Adolescent Endocrinology

Adolescent Endocrinology

Edited by
R Stanhope

Meeting supported by Serono Laboratories (UK) Ltd

Published by
BioScientifica
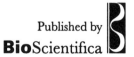

BioScientifica LTD

16 The Courtyard, Woodlands,
Bradley Stoke, Bristol BS32 4NQ, UK

©1998 BioScientifica Ltd

British Library Cataloguing in Publication Data
A CIP catalogue record for this book is available from the British Library.

ISBN 1 901978 01 X

Disclaimer

The papers contained in this book have been prepared and written by a medical writer based on oral presentations by the named authors. Accordingly, neither BioScientifica Ltd, Serono Laboratories, (UK) Ltd nor their officers, employees or agents are responsible for the accuracy or otherwise of any papers and shall have no liability for any claims, damages or losses however arising from the contents of any papers or use to which they may be put by any person.

Printed in Great Britain by J W Arrowsmith Ltd, Bristol

Foreword

Perhaps paediatric endocrinology is more aligned to adult endocrinology than to paediatrics. Unfortunately, the interface between paediatric and adult endocrinology, especially with regard to pubertal induction and the onset of fertility, is not often practised in a cohesive fashion. Indeed, modern training schedules in paediatric endocrinology do not usually encourage joint training in both specialities. There are many diseases which are thought of as the remit of adult endocrinology, such as polycystic ovary syndrome and osteoporosis, but we are beginning to realise that these are disorders of childhood and adolescence, which are expressed in adult life.

For two decades, my predominant interest has revolved around pubertal maturation and I was delighted when Serono UK allowed me to be the convenor of a meeting on adolescent endocrinology, which was held in Cambridge in December 1996; this formed the catalyst for this publication. Instead of authors submitting formal chapters, which may have had little reference to the lecture they had given, we have tried to retain the freshness of the meeting by using transcripts of the lectures, which were subsequently modified by the authors. These have been compiled into this short book which I hope will be easily digested. The aim was not to produce a textbook, but an interesting account of the subject, with a few key references for further reading.

I am indebted to Serono UK, who provided the organisation and secretarial help for the whole meeting. The setting of Queen's College, Cambridge, could not have been more outstanding even in the middle of an English winter. I was fortunate in having an enthusiastic team of colleagues who formed the scientific committee: Dr J Bevan, Consultant Endocrinologist, Aberdeen Royal Infirmary; Dr P Bouloux, Consultant Endocrinologist, Royal Free Hospital, London; Dr P Clayton, Consultant Paediatric Endocrinologist, Royal Manchester Children's Hospital, Manchester; Dr G Conway, Consultant Endocrinologist, The Middlesex Hospital, London; Dr D Dunger, Consultant Paediatric Endocrinologist, John Radcliffe Hospital, Oxford and Dr R Ross, Consultant Endocrinologist, Northern General Hospital, Sheffield. The contribution from the scientific committee formed the structure for the meeting, and their able chairmanship of the various sessions harmonised the programme into more of a workshop than a conference. I am grateful to them for their ideas and encouragement.

I am particularly grateful to Professor I Hughes, Professor of Paediatrics at Addenbrooke's Hospital, Cambridge, who not only contributed to the scientific programme, but also helped with local aspects of the meeting. I hope this book is some reflection of the originality and enthusiasm of the Cambridge meeting.

Richard Stanhope
Great Ormond Street Hospital for Children and The Middlesex Hospital (UCLH) London, UK

Contents

Endocrinology and the new genetics

3   Puberty and the new genetics
     J S Parks

Optimal hormone replacement

11   Can growth hormone change bone mass in adolescence?
     Y Seino

17   Growth hormone replacement in young adults: if and when to continue?
     D G Johnston, K A S Al-Shoumer, S A Beshyah,
     A Chrisoulidou, E Kousta and V Anyaoku

25   Oestrogen and progestogen replacement
     H S Jacobs

Puberty and fertility

33   Ovarian development: from foetus to adult
     I Huhtaniemi

39   Menarche
     M Rees

45   Gonadotrophic requirements for ovulation in adolescent girls
     D Baird

51   Outlook for males with hypogonadotrophic hypogonadism
     M Vandeweghe

59   Management of infertility and the newer reproductive techniques:
     treatment opportunities and ethical implications
     M C Davies

Virilisation and psychosexual adjustment

71   Psychosexual development of women with congenital adrenal
     hyperplasia
     K J Zucker

The adrenal, the ovary and hirsutism

79   The clinical spectrum of congenital adrenal hyperplasia in adolescence
     and adulthood
     R Azziz

85   Long-term sequelae of premature adrenarche and pubarche
     L Ibáñez and N Potau

93   Hirsutism and irregular menses in adolescence
     E Porcu and S Venturoli

101 Is polycystic ovary a condition of childhood?
     G S Conway

Weight- and exercise-related endocrine disorders

107 The control of fat mass: insights from mouse genetics
     S O'Rahilly and S Farooqi

113 Weight and reproductive endocrine dysfunction
     S Franks

119 Anabolic steroid and associated drug misuse
     A R W Forrest

125 Author index

127 Subject index

Endocrinology and the new genetics

Adolescent Endocrinology
Ed R Stanhope
BioScientifica Ltd, Bristol (1998)

Puberty and the new genetics

J S Parks

Division of Pediatric Endocrinology, Emory University School of
Medicine, Atlanta, Georgia, USA

This chapter reviews some of the genetic mechanisms controlling hormone secretion and thereby regulating pubertal development. They may be studied on three levels. In the first, mutations of known genes in the hypothalamic/ pituitary/gonadal (HPG) axis are detected and, in the second more recent approach, linkage analysis and positional cloning are used to define new genes, the general locations of which are known. Both approaches are concerned with monogenetic causes of pubertal disorders.

The third and newest approach views pubertal development as a complex phenotype in which variations in appearance and tempo of puberty reflect normal polymorphic variations in a few contributing genes. Identifying these genes and determining their contribution to puberty requires a combination of quantitative genetic analysis, genome mapping and assessments of how candidate genes are transmitted in populations and contribute to the phenotype.

Mutations of known genes in the HPG axis

Figure 1 summarizes some of the mutations that affect the luteinizing hormone (LH)/follicle-stimulating hormone (FSH) axis. Different mutations in several of these genes can cause absent, incomplete, or premature puberty. At each level, candidate genes have been identified and associated with specific developmental anomalies. At the hypothalamic level, they involve Dax-1, steroidogenesis factor-1 (SF-1) and LH-releasing hormone (LHRH). Candidate genes at the pituitary gonadotrope level are the LHRH receptor, Dax-1 and SF-1, and genes for the β-subunits of LH and FSH. Gonadotrophin receptors, the G_α-stimulatory subunit (GaS), SF-1, testosterone and oestradiol synthetic enzymes are targets for mutation at the gonadal level, and steroid receptors represent points of vulnerability in target tissues. Some examples of mutations that affect pubertal development follow.

The hyp mouse and Kallmann's syndrome

These are good genetic models of the hypogonadotrophic hypogonadism phenotype, in which puberty is absent. In the hyp mouse, gonadotrophin-releasing hormone (GnRH) neurones are present in the hypothalamus, but deletions of exons 3 and 4 of the structural GnRH gene lead to defective

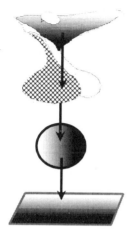

Fig. 1 Some mutations affecting the LH/FSH axis

mRNA. By contrast, in Kallmann's syndrome of humans, GnRH neurones are absent, and gene localization studies have shown that the abnormal product is a protein necessary for the normal migration and function of the hypothalamic neurones: KAL-X ECM (Kallman-X chromosome extracellular matrix) adhesion protein. The candidate gene for the non-X-linked type of Kallmann's syndrome is not yet known.

Abnormal LH or FSH β–glycoprotein hormone subunits
Homozygosity for a mis-sense inactivating mutation in codon 54, with arginine replaced by glutamic acid (Glu54Arg), affects the human LH-β gene on chromosome 19 and causes hypogonadism with high LH levels but low LH activity. Male heterozygotes are infertile (1). A mutation at codon 61 (11p13, a deletion of 2 bp and consequent frameshift) inactivates the structural gene for FSH on the short (p) arm of chromosome 11 causing amenorrhoea in homozygotes (2).

Abnormal LH receptor
The LH receptor is affected by both inactivating and activating mutations, affecting principally the sixth of seven membrane-spanning domains. Inactivating mutations are associated with failure of pubertal development, so that females appear normal at birth, but genetic males are prenatally undervirilized. High values of immunoassay and bioactivity for LH are present, together with low testosterone in males. One such inactivating mutation is an

Ala593Pro mutation on 2p21 in which LH binds normally to the receptor but there is no activation of G-protein and adenylate cyclase. The phenotype has undervirilization and lack of pubertal progression (3).

Activating mutations have been associated with male-limited precocious puberty, with onset of autonomous testicular activity and rapid virilization below the age of 4 years. High testosterone and low LH and FSH show that this process is gonadotrophin-independent. Of the possible activating mutations, Asp578Gly is the most common in the USA, and others include Met398Thr, Ile542Leu, Asp564Gly and Asp578Tyr. Expressing the protein in target cells reveals increased basal cAMP production and a variable response to LH (3-8). The sequence during puberty is evidently as follows: gonadotrophin-independent testosterone production during early childhood induces early maturation of the HPG axis. With an increase in LH and FSH production, there is a further increase in testosterone production and growth of tubular elements in addition to Leydig cells.

Linkage analysis and positional cloning to define new genes: the 'new genetics'

Adrenal hypoplasia congenita with hypogonadotrophic hypogonadism (AHC + HG) is a relatively common (1/10 000) X-linked monogenic disorder that may be part of a contiguous gene syndrome including Duchenne muscular dystrophy and glycerol kinase deficiency. The gene responsible for AHC has been localized to a critical region on the short arm of the X chromosome (9). This Dax-1 gene encodes a transcriptional regulatory protein. It is expressed in GnRH nuclei, in pituitary gonadotrophs, and in the adrenal cortex. Its levels are regulated by SF-1. Mutations of this gene cause AHC by developmental failure of the adrenal cortex, and HHG by abnormal function of GnRH nuclei and gonadotropes (at both of which the defect is probably expressed) (10, 11).

Complex phenotypes: the 'newest genetics'

In order to analyse the third category of genetic variations (i.e. those responsible for complex phenotypes, also known as polygenic, oligogenic, or multifactorial), collections of large kindreds are needed. To these, the advanced techniques of candidate gene approach, genome mapping and complex segregation analysis can be applied to assess the contributions of specific chromosomal loci to the phenotype.

Monogenic disorders and complex phenotypes

Table 1 distinguishes the major characteristics of monogenic disorders and complex phenotypes. Looking at data on 11-12-year-old children in the USA (7th grade) illustrates some specific genetic influence on development.

Table 1 Monogenic disorders, complex phenotypes, and puberty

Monogenic disorders	Complex phenotypes
Rare - 1/10 000 - 1/1 000 000 (1% of live births)	Common to universal
Individuals and sometimes their families must be studied	To examine genetic contributions, collections of large kindreds are needed
Linkage within a pedigree is analysed by simple Lod score	Heritability of particular traits can then be estimated
	Linkage analysis indicates the extent to which a particular locus contributes to heritability

Functional significance of polymorphisms in LH-β

There is a functionally important polymorphism in the gene encoding the human LH-β subunit. The less common allele, with a gene frequency of about 15%, encodes arginine rather than tryptophan at residue 8, and threonine rather than isoleucine at residue 15. It results in an LH molecule with subtly altered immunoreactivity, circulating half-life and biological activity.

Rajkhowa *et al.* (12) found that this polymorphism was not associated with polycystic ovary syndrome, although it was more frequent in obese patients with this syndrome. Hormone levels (testosterone, oestradiol and sex-hormone-binding globulin) were higher in controls with than without polymorphism. A longitudinal study of 49 Finnish boys by Raivio *et al.* (13) found that those with the polymorphism had consistently lower testicular volumes and slower growth than those without.

Thus the less common LH-β allele seems to be associated with reduced height in childhood, although it is still debatable whether the data reflect a delay in onset or a slower progression through puberty. In addition, there may be a reduction in adult height. Further issues relating to this candidate gene and its polymorphism are its impact on adult height, a quantitative genetic analysis and its interaction with other loci.

Summary

Mutations in the LH and FSH axis can cause disease. Some of these diseases result in too little sex hormone, and some can be associated with loss of function, gain of function or premature function. In the future, a host of other genes will probably also be found to influence normal progression through puberty.

References

1   Weiss J, Axelrod L, Whitcomb RW, Harris PE, Crowley WF & Jameson JL. Hypogonadism caused by a single amino acid substitution in the beta subunit of luteinizing hormone. *New England Journal of Medicine* 1992 **326** 179-183.

2   Matthews CH, Borgato S, Beck-Peccoz P, Adams M, Tone Y, Gambino G, Casagraude S, Tedeschini G, Benedetti A, & Chatterjee VK. Primary amenorrhoea and infertility due to a mutation of the beta-subunit of follicle-stimulating hormone. *Nature Genetics* 1993 **5** 83-86.

3   Kremer H, Kraaij R, Toledo SP, Post M, Fridman JB, Hayashida CY, van Reen M, Milgrom E, Ropers HH, Mariman E *et al.* Male pseudohermaphroditism due to a homozygous missense mutation of the luteinizing hormone receptor gene. *Nature Genetics* 1995 **9** 160-164.

4   Shenker A, Laue L, Kosugi S, Merendino JJ Tr, Minegishi T & Cutler GB Jr. A constitutively activating mutation of the luteinizing hormone receptor in familial male precocious puberty. *Nature* 1993 **365** 652-654.

5   Yano K, Saji M, Hidaka A, Moriya N, Okuno A, Kohn LD & Cutler GB Jr. A new constitutively activating point mutation in the luteinizing hormone/ choriogonadotropin receptor gene in cases of male-limited precocious puberty. *Journal of Clinical Endocrinology and Metabolism* 1995 **80** 1162-1168.

6   Latronico AC, Anasti J, Arnhold IJ, Mendonca BB, Domenice S, Albano MC, Zachman K, Wajchenburg BL, & Tsigos C. A novel mutation of the luteinizing hormone receptor gene causing male gonadotropin-independent precocious puberty. *Journal of Clinical Endocrinology and Metabolism* 1995 **80** 2490-2494.

7   Kraaij R, Post M, Kremer H, Mulgrom E, Epping W, Brunner HG, Grootegoer JA, & Themmen AP. A missense mutation in the second transmembrane segment of the luteinizing hormone receptor causes familial male-limited precocious puberty. *Journal of Clinical Endocrinology and Metabolism* 1996 **80** 3168-3172.

8   Themmen AP & Brunner HG. Luteinizing hormone receptor mutations and sex differentiation. *European Journal of Endocrinology* 1996 **134** 533-540.

9   Zanaria E, Muscatelli F, Bardoni B, Strom TM, Guioli S, Guo W, Lalli E, Moser C, Walker AP, McCabe ER, *et al.* An unusual member of the nuclear hormone receptor superfamily responsible for X-linked adrenal hypoplasia congenita. *Nature* 1994 **372** 635-641.

10   Muscatelli F, Strom TM, Walker AP, Zanaria E, Recan D, Meindl A, Bardoni B, Guioli S, Zehetner G, Rabl W, *et al.* Mutations in the DAX-1 gene give rise to both X-linked adrenal hypoplasia congenita and hypogonadotropic hypogonadism. *Nature* 1994 **372** 672-676.

11   Suganuma N, Furui K, Kikkawa F, Tomoda Y & Furuhashi M. Effects of the mutations (Trp8 → Arg and Ile15 → Thr) in human luteinizing hormone (LH) beta-subunit on LH bioactivity in vitro and in vivo. *Endocrinology* 1996 **137** 831-838.

12   Rajkhowa M, Talbot JA, Jones PW, Petterson K, Haavisto AM, Huhtaniemi I & Clayton RN. Prevalence of an immunological LH beta-subunit variant in a UK population of healthy women and women with polycystic ovary syndrome. *Clinical Endocrinology* 1995 **43** 297-303.

13   Raivio T, Huhtaniemi I, Anttila R, Siimes MA, Hagenas L, Nilsson C, Petterson K & Dunkel L. The role of luteinizing hormone-beta gene polymorphism in the onset and progression of puberty in healthy boys. *Journal of Clinical Endocrinology and Metabolism* 1996 **81** 3278-3282.

Optimal hormone replacement

Adolescent Endocrinology
Ed R Stanhope
BioScientifica Ltd, Bristol (1998)

Can growth hormone change bone mass in adolescence?

Y Seino

Department of Paediatrics, Okayama Medical School, Okayama,
Japan

Bone growth during childhood is critically important for achieving adequate bone mass in adult life. Several markers of bone metabolism, both formation and resorption, can be identified non-invasively in the serum and urine. This paper describes changes in bone metabolism and bone mass during adolescence using metabolic markers and X-ray absorptiometry, and reports how growth hormone (GH)-deficient children can achieve significant bone growth during GH therapy.

Bone growth and osteoporosis

In osteoporosis the trabecular architecture of bone is destroyed. This disease is becoming increasingly serious world wide. Osteoporotic fractures consign elderly people to bed and, in Japan alone, the number affected will reach 10 million by 2001.

Peak bone mass (PBM)

There are two ways of preventing osteoporosis. Preventing loss of bone mass has long been considered the more important form of protection from osteoporosis, but it is now being recognized that increasing PBM is another key to prevention. A decrease in bone mass of 3 standard deviations from mean peak height will cause 90% of fractures. In people with a high PBM, the osteoporotic fracture risk level will not be reached during the normal decline in bone mass density (BMD), whereas a lower PBM means a definite risk.

Japanese national survey of osteoporosis

I am currently conducting a nationwide measurement of PBM in Japan, and Figure 1 shows cross-sectional data on females from 3 to 90 years of age. PBM is represented by a BMD of 1.0. In women, PBM is maintained up to age 45, while in men it begins to decline only after age 70, so that osteoporosis is predominantly a women's disease.

In 1994 Matkovic *et al.* reported that in the USA BMD achieved in late adolescence continues at a constant level for up to 50 years (1). Similar findings apply to Australia (2). The message is that, world wide, PBM develops during adolescence.

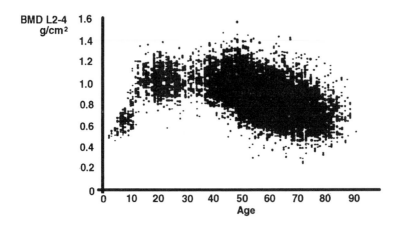

Fig. 1 BMD in females aged 3-90 in the Japanese population. n=13191

Bone growth rate (BGR)

BGR indicates how much BMD increases over time (analogously to height velocity). In Japan, BGR peaks in females at 12-13 years, and in males at 13-14 years (3). Swiss data from Bonjour and colleagues show the same picture with respect to both lumbar spine and femur neck; most importantly, they also demonstrate that no further bone accumulated in any area of the skeleton studied after age 20 (4).

About 40% of bone mass accumulates between Tanner pubertal stages 2 and 4, and so, in terms of prevention, osteoporosis can be considered a paediatric not a geriatric disease.

Bone formation during adolescence

The interaction between sex hormones, GH and growth factors is responsible for accumulating bone. The two major modes of bone growth, elongation and thickening, are greatly accelerated during adolescence. Enchondral bone formation results in elongation, and osteomembranous ossification results in thickening. The slope of the standard height-velocity curve is highest in infancy and adolescence, showing that bone growth also peaks at these periods.

Key factors operating through hormones to affect bone gain are:

Genetics: e.g. defects in receptors for vitamin D, oestrogen, or other growth factors

Nutritional state: particularly calcium intake (anorexia nervosa is associated with very low bone density)

Exercise: astronauts living in microgravity experience significant bone loss.

Table 1 Metabolic markers of bone formation and resorption

Bone formation
  Serum osteocalcin
  Serum type 1 collagen (P1CP)
  Serum bone alkaline phosphatase

Bone resorption
  Serum type 1 collagen cross-linked C-telopeptide (1CTP)
  Serum tartrate-resistant acid phosphatase (TRAP)
  Urinary pyridinoline, deoxypyridinoline (PYR, DPYR)
  Urinary hydroxyproline
  Urinary type 1 collagen cross-linked N-telopeptide (1NTP)

Metabolic bone markers

Table 1 lists some important metabolic markers of bone mineralization.

Bone remodelling consists of osteoclasts breaking down bone for a few weeks followed by osteoblasts making bone day by day. Osteocalcin is a peptide produced only by osteoblasts. It is metabolized from prepro-osteocalcin via pro-osteocalcin, but some osteocalcin is also incorporated into bone matrix before mineralization. Again, when bone is degraded, osteocalcin is also secreted, so its level is high in states of both bone formation and bone resorption (Fig. 2) (5).

Levels of osteocalcin and serum bone alkaline phosphatase are high in both infancy and adolescence, and their levels parallel the height-velocity curve.

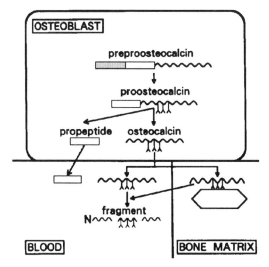

Fig. 2 Some aspects of bone formation. Reproduced with permission from (5) © The Endocrine Society

Metabolism of type 1 collagen

Type 1 collagen is the most abundant bone matrix protein. When osteoblasts are activated, procollagen type 1 is secreted and releases N-terminal or C-terminal telopeptide (1CTP, 1NTP) to leave type 1 collagen (P1CP). Molecules of type 1 collagen become cross-linked by pyridinoline/deoxypyridinoline (PYR/DPYR). Thus levels of P1CP in the blood reflect the rate of bone formation.

Conversely, when bone is degraded, P1CP releases 1CTP or 1NTP into the blood, so serum 1CTP reflects the rate of bone degradation. In addition, levels of PYR or DPYR secreted into the urine also indicate the rate of bone degradation (Table 1). PYR is present in both cartilage and bone, whereas DPYR, being found only in bone, is the more specific marker.

Like levels of osteocalcin and serum bone alkaline phosphatase, the bone formation marker P1CP and the degradation marker 1CTP are also high during infancy and adolescence. In addition, PYR and DPYR levels are constantly high during the growing period, rising further in adolescence.

Figure 3 illustrates annual BGR, together with levels of alkaline phosphatase and osteocalcin before and during puberty. Levels of these bone formation markers rise about 2 years before BGR increases, suggesting that they can be used to predict bone growth. However, levels of PYR and DPYR merely stay constantly high, declining rapidly after puberty.

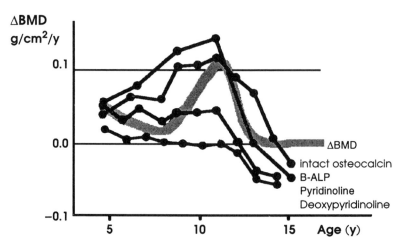

Fig. 3 Annual BGR and levels of alkaline phosphatase (B-ALP) osteocalcin, PYR, and DPYR before and during puberty.

Effects of GH

Serum levels of the bone formation markers osteocalcin, bone alkaline phosphatase and propeptide increase for the first 6 months after treatment with GH, and bone resorption is also enhanced, as shown by increases in markers such as DPYR and PYR. In addition, the bone resorption marker 1CTP increases rapidly and remains high after treatment, whereas the formation marker P1CP (type 1 collagen) increases gradually up to 6 months; perhaps treatment stimulates first bone breakdown and then formation.

P1CP metabolism and GH

When bone is formed, P1CP is released into the blood, and, when it is degraded, 1CTP is released into the blood from type 1 collagen. These compounds are released in a 1:1 molar ratio, so their ratio may reflect the state of bone balance. This ratio does indeed gradually increase during GH treatment, indicating a positive bone balance.

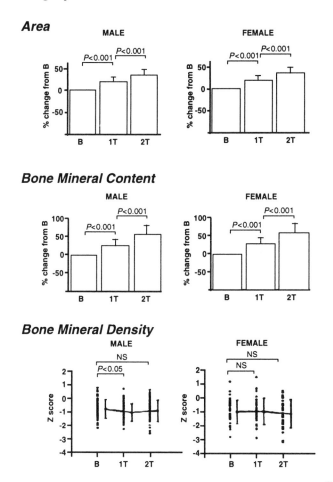

Fig. 4 Beneficial effects on height and bone parameters of GH, 2 IU/m^2 per day, in 110 GH deficient patients. B, Before therapy; 1T, 2T, 1 and 2 years after therapy respectively. Results are means±s.D.

Can GH change bone mass during adolescence?

The following are preliminary data from 2 years of experience with GH treatment in 72 males and 38 females (4-17 years of age), who were partially GH deficient (i.e. stimulated serum GH <10 ng/ml). The dose was 0.5 IU/kg per week (2 IU/m^2 per day). Lumbar spine BMD, defined as bone mineral content (BMC)/unit area, was measured by the standard method, dual-energy X-ray absorptiometry.

Effects of GH treatment

GH treatment resulted in several beneficial changes. Height increased, BMC significantly increased in both males and females (Fig. 4), and projected bone area and bone mass increased. However, BMD, as defined above, and true volumetric BMD remained constant, because BMC and bone size both increased during GH treatment.

Our interim conclusions are that GH stimulated bone growth, with an appropriate increase in bone mass in GH-deficient patients during childhood, and maintained BMD during treatment.

References

1   Matkovic V, Jelic T, Wardlaw GM, Ilich JZ, Goel PK, Wright JK, Andon MB, Smith KT & Heaney RP. Timing of peak bone mass in Caucasian females and its implication for the prevention of osteoporosis. Inference from a cross-sectional model. *Journal of Clinical Investigation* 1994 **93** 799-808.

2   Lu PW, Briody JN, Ogle GD, Morley K, Humphries IR, Allen J, Howman-Giles R, Sillence D & Cowell CT. Bone mineral density of total body, spine, and femoral neck in children and young adults: a cross-sectional and longitudinal study. *Journal of Bone and Mineral Research* 1994 **9** 1451-1458.

3   Seino Y, Tanaka H, Fukunaga M, Nishiyama S, Hirota T, Fukuoka H, Orimo H & Matsuda I. Bone growth in Japanese children : Peak bone mass and environmental factors. In: *Frontiers in Endocrinology 17: Sexual Differentiation and Maturation*, pp 239-243. Eds I Hibi & T Tanaka. London: Ares-Serono Symposia Publications, 1996.

4   Bonjour JP, Theintz G, Buchs B, Slosman D & Rizzoli R. Critical years and stages of puberty for spinal and femoral bone mass accumulation during adolescence. *Journal of Clinical Endocrinology and Metabolism* 1991 **73** 555-563.

5   Kanzaki S, Hosoda K, Moriwake T, Tanaka H, Kubo T, Inoue M, Higuchi J, Yamaji T & Seino Y. Serum propeptide and intact molecular osteocalcin in normal children and children with growth hormone (GH) deficiency: a potential marker of bone growth and response to GH therapy. *Journal of Clinical Endocrinology and Metabolism* 1992 **75** 1104-1109.

Growth hormone replacement in young adults: if and when to continue?

D G Johnston, K A S Al-Shoumer, S A Beshyah, A Chrisoulidou, E Kousta and V Anyaoku

Unit of Metabolic Medicine, Imperial College School of Medicine,
St Mary's Hospital, Praed Street, London, UK

As in many areas of medicine, the questions in the title of this chapter cannot be answered without undertaking an impractical study on a large cohort of young patients who have been treated with growth hormone (GH) in childhood with the aim of enhancing growth; half will need to be treated with GH after growth has ceased, and their outcomes compared with those of the untreated half 50 years later. A judgment based on the available evidence is as much as can practically be done.

Hypopituitarism in adulthood

What has been achieved in hypopituitary patients who have and have not received GH treatment?

Excess mortality

A well-known Swedish study (1) examined the data on 104 patients who had died out of 333 hypopituitary patients diagnosed between 1956 and 1987 and who had not received GH. Actuarial data predicted only half the total mortality found (actuarial 57 vs 104 actual), and vascular disease was an important source of excess mortality (31 vs 60). Other studies have since confirmed the excess of vascular deaths in these patients (2, 3).

The study of Bulow *et al.* (3) found that most of the excess vascular disease was cerebrovascular, and that its frequency was greater in women than in men.

Prompted by these findings, my colleagues and I looked for evidence of vascular disease during life in our hypopituitary patients at St Mary's Hospital, London. The number of atheromatous plaques was counted, and the intima-media thickness in the carotid and femoral arteries determined by high-resolution B-mode ultrasound imaging (4, 5).

Peripheral arterial disease and hypopituitarism

Intima-media thickness in the carotid arteries is a particularly important measure because it correlates with vascular disease elsewhere in the body and with other risk factors (e.g. coronary artery disease, smoking, hypercholesterolaemia). We found that, compared with non-hypopituitary controls ($n=29$), hypopituitary patients in their middle and later years ($n=28$) had significantly elevated mean intima-media thickness (4).

- 40-60 years; 0.72 vs 0.64mm ($P<0.02$)
- >60 years: 0.90 vs 0.80mm ($P<0.05$)

In the same study, the proportion of subjects who had one atheromatous plaque or more was significantly higher among hypopituitary patients than among controls: 65 vs 41% *(P<0.05)*. As vascular disease develops, arteries become less distensible, more compliant and stiffer; these changes were also greater in the hypopituitary patients than controls. Thus the distensibility coefficient was decreased ($24.2\,(\pm2.3)\times10^{-3}$ *vs* $30.1\,(\pm2.0)\times10^{-3}$ kPa^{-1}; $P<0.05$), the compliance coefficient was decreased ($5.7\,(\pm0.5)\times10^{-7}$ *vs* $7.0\,(\pm0.5)\times10^{-7}$ kPa^{-1}; $P<0.05$) and the beta index (a measure of arterial wall stiffness) was increased (8.4 ± 1.3 vs 5.9 ± 0.4; $P<0.05$) in 34 hypopituitary adults compared with 39 matched controls (5).

So there is evidence that hypopituitary patients not only die young, but also have an excess of vascular disease during life.

The heart and hypopituitarism (6)

Echocardiographic and treadmill exercise tests performed on the hypopituitary patients revealed changes that may indicate very early stages of ischaemic heart disease. Echocardiography revealed abnormalities in diastolic function (e.g. isovolumic relaxation time) in 9/39 patients, and evidence of S-T segment depression on the electrocardiogram was seen in 12/39.

Aetiologies of vascular disease

A variety of mechanisms can be responsible for the development of vascular disease, including:

- anthropometric features
- hyperglycaemia/hyperinsulinaemia
- blood-clotting abnormalities
- lipid/lipoprotein abnormalities

Lipid and lipoprotein abnormalities in hypopituitary patients

Table 1 summarizes some lipid parameters in our hypopituitary patients and non-hypopituitary controls, together with some anthropometric and demographic data (7). Controls were matched for age, sex and body mass index.

Waist/hip ratio was significantly greater in hypopituitary patients than in controls (0.879 vs 0.830; $P=0.0005$), consistent with the type of central body fat distribution normally associated with increased prevalence of coronary artery disease. Likewise, serum total cholesterol, triglycerides and low-density lipoprotein (LDL)-cholesterol levels were all elevated in hypopituitary patients relative to controls; these are all changes associated with premature vascular

Table 1 Some demographic and anthropometric data, and circulating fasting lipid concentrations in hypopituitary patients and non-hypopituitary controls (full details are provided in reference (7)). Results are means±S.E.M.

Parameter	Patients	Controls	P
Number	67	87	-
Sex (M/F)	31/36	33/45	-
Age (years)	48±2	45±1	-
Body mass index (kg/m^2)	28.1±0.6	27.1±0.6	-
Waist/hip ratio	0.879±0.012	0.830±0.009	0.0005
Lipids (mmol/l)			
Total cholesterol	6.44±0.19	5.73±0.16	0.017
Triglyceride	1.75±0.15	1.39±0.09	0.19
HDL-colesterol	1.20±0.15	1.26±0.05	0.004
LDL-cholesterol	4.53±0.19	3.89±0.15	0.0005

disease; however, as in many other studies, high-density lipoprotein (HDL)-cholesterol levels were not depressed.

These abnormalities predominated in women, and changes in men were much less. The cause of this difference is difficult to understand; it did not simply correlate with sex-hormone replacement therapy. The dyslipidaemias found in the hypopituitary patients affected not only the fasting state but also the postprandial state; once again the changes were most marked in women. So, with regard to lipid disorders in hypopituitary adults, we conclude that:

- lipid disorders are common
- total cholesterol, LDL-cholesterol and triglycerides are elevated
- the dyslipidaemia affects women irrespective of the need for hormone replacement therapy

The causative mechanisms of the dyslipidaemia are not well understood, but inappropriate use of glucocorticoid, thyroid hormones or sex hormones could be involved (7).

Glucose tolerance and diabetes

In this middle-aged overweight population of 62 hypopituitary patients, 20 (32%) were found to have impaired glucose tolerance, and seven (11%) had diabetes, about twice the prevalences found in a comparable non-hypopituitary group in the general population (8). Diabetes and impaired glucose tolerance are also, of course, risk factors for cardiovascular disease. Even in the hypopituitary patients without diabetes, mean blood glucose and insulin were somewhat elevated after the oral glucose tolerance test.

No difference was found between patients and controls with respect to blood clot formation or lysis, although other workers have found elevated plasma fibrinogen and other abnormalities (9).

GH in hypopituitary patients

Insulin levels

Our ongoing study of the effects of GH in hypopituitary adults (10) showed that, after 6 months of treatment, their fasting plasma insulin and C-peptide levels increased relative to controls (Table 2). Not only intact proinsulin but also 32-33 split proinsulin increased over 6 months; work in Cambridge (11) has shown that these changes characterize insulin resistance and may be early signs of β-cell failure.

Table 2 Effects of therapy on fasting plasma glucose, insulin and C-peptide levels (full details are provided in reference (8)).

	Concentration (mmol/l)			
	GH-treated		**Placebo-treated**	
Parameter	Baseline	6 months	Baseline	6 months
Glucose (mean±s.d.)	4.9±0.8	5.2±0.6	4.7±0.4	4.8±0.7
Insulin (median and range)	17 (0-91)	58 (14-335)**	22 (0-235)	36 (0-190)
C-peptide (median and range)	530 (166-2152)	794 (132-1357)*	497 (331-1456)	497 (364-1324)

*$P<0.05$, **$P<0.01$ compared with baseline.

Glucose tolerance

Treatment with GH for 6 months produced mild hyperglycaemia and more marked hyperinsulinaemia in the hypopituitary patients. Available data on our patients who have received GH for up to 4 years show that fasting hyperglycaemia disappeared with prolonged treatment, but hyperinsulinaemia persisted; in addition, hyperglycaemia induced by the oral glucose tolerance test diminished over time, but stimulated hyperinsulinaemia remained equivocal.

Lipid parameters in hypopituitary patients treated with GH

GH treatment was highly beneficial in terms of lipid profile and hence cardiovascular risk. A significant decline in total cholesterol concentration ($P<0.02$) seen after 12 months of GH treatment persisted over the full 4 years of treatment, and LDL-cholesterol also decreased. Triglyceride and HDL-cholesterol levels did not change. A significant decrease in waist/hip ratio at 12 months (P=0.005) was also sustained over the following 3 years of treatment (P=0.024, 0.05, 0.03) (12).

Long-term studies need controls, but a long-term placebo control group is not now an option; therefore we are currently assembling an historical group of hypopituitary individuals whose lipid profiles, body composition, glucose homoeostasis and insulin sensitivity were documented in the late 1980s, but who received little or no GH treatment.

GH treatment and mortality
This chapter has focused on vascular disease because one concern in terms of mortality in hypopituitary patients is premature death from vascular disease. It is not yet clear whether GH treatment will influence this premature mortality, but it can now be said that GH has beneficial effects in terms of body composition and lipid lowering, but that increases in fasting insulin and intact and split proinsulin would normally be considered non-beneficial.

Advantages and disadvantages of continuing GH treatment in adult life
There are many other reasons to continue GH treatment in adulthood after treating the hypopituitary child. Aspects of quality of life are diminished in GH-deficient young people, particularly as a result of their short stature. Studies have shown that quality of life is also impaired in hypopituitarism compared with the general population, although the same probably applies to any chronic illness and not necessarily hypopituitarism *per se*. We have found that quality of life in these patients was lower than that in those with non-insulin-dependent diabetes (13), although an Oxford study showed no difference in comparison with patients undergoing mastoid surgery (14). Most studies show that quality of life in these patients improves with GH treatment (15). There are other reasons to continue GH therapy. For example, GH can increase muscle power (16). We and others have demonstrated an improvement in exercise tolerance with prolonged GH treatment (6). At least with long-term replacement therapy, GH has beneficial effects on bone mineral density which may reduce the risk of osteoporosis in later life (17).

The disadvantages of continuing GH treatment are obvious: it is expensive, involves daily injections and may have certain adverse metabolic effects. Whether long-term treatment may increase the incidence of certain tumours, causing disorders such as bowel polyps or frank neoplasia, for example, is not yet known. Years of monitoring large numbers will be needed to answer such questions.

Conclusion
In summary, there is conflicting evidence on many points relating to whether and when to treat young hypopituitary adults with GH, so for the present clinicians must come to treatment decisions for each individual patient. With

more experience, optimum dosage regimens may be developed which will maximize the benefits and minimize the risks. We may also become better at selecting for treatment those patients who will benefit most.

References

1   Rosén T & Bengtsson B-A. Premature mortality due to cardiovascular disease in hypopituitarism. *Lancet* 1990 **336** 285-288.

2   Wüster C, Slenczka E & Ziegler R. Increased prevalence of osteoporosis and arteriosclerosis in conventionally substituted anterior pituitary insufficiency: need for additional growth hormone substitution? *Klinische Wochenschrifte* 1991 **69** 769-773.

3   Bulow B, Hagman L, Mikoczy Z, Nordstrom CH & Erfurth EM. Increased cerebrovascular mortality in patients with hypopituitarism. *Clinical Endocrinology* 1997 **46** 75-81.

4   Markussis V, Beshyah SA, Fisher C, Sharp P, Nicolaides AN & Johnston DG. Detection of premature atherosclerosis by high-resolution ultrasonography in symptom-free hypopituitary adults. *Lancet* 1992 **340** 1188-1192.

5   Markussis V, Beshyah SA, Fisher C, Parker KH, Nicolaides AN & Johnston DG. Abnormal carotid arterial wall dynamics in symptom-free hypopituitary adults. *European Journal of Endocrinology* 1997 **136** 157-164.

6   Shahi M, Beshyah SA, Hackett D, Sharp PS, Johnston DG & Foale RA. Myocardial dysfunction in treated adult hypopituitarism: a possible explanation for increased cardiovascular mortality. *British Heart Journal* 1992 **67** 92-96.

7   Al-Shoumer KAS, Cox K, Hughes C, Richmond W & Johnston DG. Fasting and post-prandial lipid abnormalities in hypopituitary women on conventional replacement therapy. *Journal of Clinical Endocrinology and Metabolism* 1997 **82** 2653-2659.

8   Beshyah SA, Henderson A, Nithyananthan R, Sharp P, Richmond W & Johnston DG. Metabolic abnormalities in growth hormone-deficient adults. II. Carbohydrate tolerance and lipid metabolism. *Endocrinology and Metabolism* 1994 **1** 173-180.

9   Johansson JO, Landin K, Tengborn L, Rosen T & Bengtsson BA. High fibrinogen and plasminogen activator inhibitor activity in growth hormone-deficient adults. *Arteriosclerosis and Thrombosis* 1994 **14** 434-437.

10 Beshyah SA, Gelding SV, Andres C, Johnston DG & Gray IP. β-cell function in hypopituitary adults before and during growth hormone treatment. *Clinical Science* 1995 **89** 321-328.

11 Temple RC, Carrington CA, Luzio SD, Owens DR, Schneider AE & Sobey WJ. Insulin deficiency in non-insulin-dependent diabetes. *Lancet* **i** 293-295.

12 Al-Shoumer KAS, Page B, Thomas E, Murphy M, Beshyah SA & Johnston DG. Effect of four years' treatment with biosynthetic growth hormone (GH). *European Journal of Endocrinology* 1996 **135** 559-567.

13 Lynch S, Merson S, Beshyah SA, Skinner E, Sharp P, Priest RG *et al.* Psychiatric morbidity in adults with hypopituitarism. *Journal of the Royal Society of Medicine* 1994 **87** 445-447.

14 Page RCL, Hammersley MS, Burke CW & Wass JAH. An account of the quality of life of patients after treatment for non-functioning pituitary tumours. *Clinical Endocrinology* 1997 **46** 401-406.

15   Johnston DG. Growth hormone deficiency and quality of life in hypopituitary adults (commentary). *Clinical Endocrinology* 1997 **46** 407-408.

16   Rutherford OM, Jones DA, Round JM, Buchanan CR & Preece MA. Changes in skeletal muscle and body composition after dicontinuation of growth hormone treatment in growth hormone deficient young adults. *Clinical Endocrinology* 1991 **34** 469-475.

17   Shalet SM. Growth hormone deficiency and replacement in adults (editorial). *British Medical Journal* 1996 **313** 314.

Oestrogen and progestogen replacement

H S Jacobs

UCL Medical School, The Middlesex Hospital, Mortimer Street,
London, UK

In view of the fact that oestrogen and progestogen replacement may have to begin in early life and continue for many years, the lack of hard evidence about hormone replacement therapy (HRT) in adolescence is staggering; most studies are observational, and few of the drugs discussed here are licensed for use in this age group. Our arguments in this field are therefore pursued by analogy with HRT in postmenopausal women, by intuition, and by experience. HRT is given to young people for delayed or absent puberty (e.g. associated with Turner's syndrome or hypopituitarism). Its immediate advantages include the promotion of sexual maturation and the resolution of symptomatic oestrogen deficiency.

Plasma oestradiol and HRT

Many years ago we investigated plasma oestradiol levels and oestrogen deficiency in postmenopausal women at St Mary's Hospital, London (1). The women, in their 50s, had no symptoms, or flushes only, or vaginal symptoms. Plasma oestradiol levels in the last group were about half those of the other groups.

It should be noted that oestrone levels did not reflect this difference, and oestradiol levels are the usual measure of oestrogen deficiency.

The major long-term aim of HRT beginning in adolescence is to prevent complications of oestrogen deficiency, the most significant of which are osteoporosis, coronary heart disease and Alzheimer's disease.

Osteoporosis

Dr Melanie Davies's work (2) on young women with oestrogen deficiency demonstrated marked loss of vertebral bone mineral density (BMD<0.85% of normal) in those with Turner's syndrome, premature ovarian failure, hypopituitarism or hypogonadotrophic hypogonadism. These patients had often been receiving HRT for 6-7 years, but treatment had begun at around age 20, very late according to current practice.

Table 1 shows very significant increases in fracture rates among the women whose BMD was diminished as a consequence of oestrogen deficiency. Only about 5% of unaffected women had had fractures, compared with one-third of those with Turner's syndrome and nearly one-half of those with primary amenorrhoea.

Table 1 Frequency of a history of fracture among young women with oestrogen deficiency

	Unaffected	Turner's syndrome	Primary amenorrhea
Fracture history	1/19	10/22	11/33
Significance	├ – – – P=0.011 – – – ┤		
	├ – – – – – – – P=0.05 – – – – – – – ┤		

HRT and BMD

Treatment that restores oestrogen levels (e.g. HRT, an anabolic regimen where weight loss is the cause, dopamine agonist therapy in hyperprolactinaemic women) results in an increase in BMD, but rarely if ever to normal values; a permanent deficit remains (3).

To sum up, with respect to full development of the skeleton, oestrogen deficiency is harmful, while oestrogen replacement is beneficial, although rarely completely successful.

Coronary heart disease

It is only now being appreciated how significant cardiovascular disease is as a cause of morbidity and mortality in women; more than half of women die from cardiovascular disease.

Relationship of hormones to heart disease

Data on deaths/1000 in England and Wales for 1970-1974 (4) show that at all ages more men than women die of heart attacks. However, at about age 50, the mean age of menopause, the slope of the curve relating heart attack risk to age for men decreases abruptly, while that for women changes little.

It seems that the fall in relative risk is to do with a change in men rather than women, suggesting that the much-reiterated cardiovascular protective value of oestrogen replacement in women may be less certain than has been supposed.

Data such as those of Graham Colditz, an enthusiastic proponent of the protective effect (5), bear re-examination. For example, the risk of non-fatal myocardial infarction/fatal heart disease appears to be significantly raised in post- relative to pre-menopausal women adjusted for 5-year age categories (relative risk 1.7). However, taking the same data set in 1-year categories abolishes the significance of the differences; and adjusting for cigarette smoking in addition to 1-year categories abolishes the differences themselves.

Thus the notion that the menopause causes heart attacks must be continually re-examined.

On the other hand, Colditz's data clearly show that the risk of heart attack is doubled in women after ovariectomy without treatment, and restored to normal with HRT. The weakness of the evidence in a field based entirely on observational studies such as these is illustrated by the conflict between the two sets of data; no large randomized controlled clinical trials with mortality from heart attacks as the end point of the study, have yet been conducted in this area.

Various studies have suggested that the relative risk of total coronary disease or non-fatal myocardial infarction in current users of HRT is about 30-60% of that in 'never-users', and discontinuing HRT leads to an increase in relative risk. The comprehensive review of Meade & Berra (6) in the UK analysed weighted results of 12 retrospective case-control studies involving nearly 1900 patients and suggested a relative reduction in risk of death from coronary heart disease of about 25% with HRT (and that for stroke, 15%). In 10 prospective cohort studies on over 15 000 patients, risk reduction was about 20%. US workers are much more optimistic in their assessments of risk reduction achievable by HRT.

Benefit reduction by gestogens?
Fears that addition of a gestogen to oestrogen in HRT to protect the uterus might reduce the cardioprotective effect of oestrogen have not been substantiated.

Alzheimer's disease

A possible beneficial role for oestrogen in Alzheimer's disease has recently been reported (7). Oestrogen is known to have several beneficial effects on brain function; it acts positively on blood flow, cholinergic markers and nerve growth factors, and negatively on glucocorticoid-induced damage and neuronal atrophy (Fig. 1).

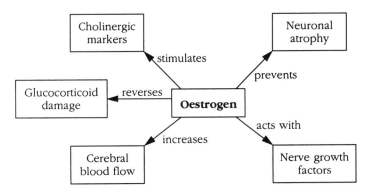

Fig. 1 Actions of oestrogen in the brain. Redrawn from (7).

Risk reduction with HRT

The Alzheimer's disease study (7) involved nearly 1000 postmenopausal women with or without HRT who were followed up for several years. Alzheimer's disease developed in 16.3% of those not using HRT, but in only 4.8% of those using HRT, representing a 60% overall risk reduction over the period of the study. The reported benefit increased considerably with longer treatment. Incidence of Alzheimer's disease was 7.5% in women who had used HRT for 1 year or less, representing a relative risk of 0.47 (confidence interval 0.20-1.10); in those using HRT for more than 1 year, relative risk fell to 0.13 (0.20-0.92), less than one-eighth of the untreated value. In this study, the onset of Alzheimer's disease was delayed rather than prevented, although it appears that treatment with oestrogen may also ameliorate the severity of the condition (8). Randomized studies are the next step in this exciting story.

Disadvantages of HRT

The disadvantages of HRT include: general problems of replacement therapy; specific problems of replacing oestrogen and progestogen (e.g. the limited range of agents and dosages available); the fear of developing cancer; important also are the increased risks of venous thrombosis/embolism and of cancer of the uterus and breast.

Venous thrombosis/embolism

A doubled causal risk of venous thrombosis/embolism is associated with HRT. This is not an automatic reason to discontinue treatment in patients with oestrogen deficiency, because there may be no alternative for them. There are, however, definite risk factors that can be identified and should be considered (e.g. obesity, varicose veins, immobility) before prescribing.

Cancer

Concern about the risk of developing cancer is the major factor limiting persistence of treatment with HRT, and must be carefully considered when very long-term hormone treatment in an adolescent patient is contemplated.

A gestogen given concurrently with oestrogen (currently with a daily dose of ethinyloestradiol of 20 µg or more, in the UK) reduces the risk of endometrial hyperplasia and cancer in both the adolescent and postmenopausal patient. At present we advise at least 14 days treatment per month with a gestogen such as norethisterone, in a dose of 2.5 mg bd.

Breast cancer is the big issue in HRT. Gestogen is not protective (9), as it is for endometrial cancer, and the risk ratio of breast cancer is about 1.3, representing a 30% increased risk of developing breast cancer with long-term (i.e. >10 years) HRT in postmenopausal women. Giving long-term (30+ years?) HRT may be exposing adolescent patients to this degree of risk, but no data on such patients are yet available. However, the presently available data strongly suggest that the risk is related to the subject's age, rather than the duration of treatment.

Postmenopausal HRT

Indications for postmenopausal HRT

In the absence of hard data, the extent to which postmenopausal indications (Table 2) might apply to an adolescent patient should be carefully considered. It is worth remembering that a calcium-deficient diet as the result of avoiding 'fattening' dairy products is probably the norm in this age group. Therefore supplementation of all regimens with the RDA of calcium should be carefully considered.

Table 2 Indications for postmenopausal HRT

Correction of the symptoms of oestrogen deficiency
    Flushing/sweating
    Vaginal/bladder symptoms
    Memory/concentration problems?

Prevention of osteoporosis - oestrogen deficiency
    Severe
    Prolonged
    Premenopausal
    Underweight
    Glucorticoid therapy
    Cigarette smoking
    Subnormal peak bone mass
    Sedentary lifestyle
    Genetic predisposition

Prevention of coronary heart disease - oestrogen deficiency
    Dyslipidaemia
    Hypertension
    Diabetes
    Cigarette smoking
    Genetic predisposition

Contraindications for postmenopausal HRT

Again, the relevance of available postmenopausal data to adolescents is uncertain. Contraindications include a history of undiagnosed vaginal bleeding, atypical endometrial hyperplasia/cancer, breast cancer, gallstones, blood-clotting deficiencies and vague psychiatric disorders.

Finally, the most important contraindication to oestrogen replacement therapy is when the patient has nothing to gain from it.

References

1   Hutton JD, Jacobs HS, Murray MAF & James VHT. Relation between plasma oestrone and oestradiol in climacteric symptoms. *Lancet* 1978 **i** 678-681.

2   Davies MC, Guleckli B & Jacobs HS. Osteoporosis in Turner's syndrome and other forms of primary amenorrhoea. *Clinical Endocrinology* 1995 **43** 741-746.

3   Guleckli B, Davies MC & Jacobs HS. Effect of treatment on established osteoporosis in young women with amenorrhoea. *Clinical Endocrinology* 1994 **41** 275-281.

4   Heller RF & Jacobs HS. Coronary heart disease in relation to age, sex, and the menopause. *British Medical Journal* 1978 **1** 424-474.

5   Colditz GA, Stampfer MJ & Willett WC. Menopause and heart disease: a review. *Annals of the New York Academy of Science* 1990 **592** 193-203.

6   Meade TW & Berra A. Hormone replacement therapy and cardiovascular disease. *British Medical Bulletin* 1992 **48** 276-308.

7   Tang MX, Jacobs D, Stern Y, Marder K, Schofield P, Gurland B, Andrews A & Mayeux R. Effect of oestrogen during menopause on risk and age of onset of Alzheimer's disease. *Lancet* 1996 **348** 429-432.

8   Ohkura T, Isse K & Akazawa K. Low-dose estrogen replacement therapy for Alzheimer's disease in women. *Menopause* 1994 **1** 125-130.

9   Colditz GA, Hankinson SE, Hunter DJ, Willett WC, Manson JE, Stampfer MJ, Hennekens C, Rosner B & Speizer FE. The use of estrogens and progestins and the risk of breast cancer in postmenopausal women. *New England Journal of Medicine* 1995 **332** 1589-1593.

Puberty and fertility

Adolescent Endocrinology
Ed R Stanhope
BioScientifica Ltd, Bristol (1998)

Ovarian development: from foetus to adult

I Huhtaniemi

Department of Physiology, Institute of Biomedicine, University of
Turku, Turku, Finland

This paper examines the two major phases of ovarian development: foetal ovarian organogenesis (morphological development) and the maturation around puberty of the cyclic ovarian function which is necessary for fertility (endocrinological development). Finally, some lessons to be learnt from studying mutations in genes for reproductive hormones are reviewed.

Ovarian morphological development

The stages of ovarian development

Table 1 outlines the stages of human ovarian development, from pregonadal cells, through an indifferent gonad, to primary and secondary sex differentiation.

The primordial germ cells differentiate in the blastocyst and migrate to the gonadal primordium in the gonadal ridge of the mesonephros. By gestational week 5-6, the three cellular components of the indifferent gonad are in place: in a future ovary, the primordial germ cells, coelomic epithelial cells, and mesenchymal cells will ultimately develop into ova, granulosa cells and stroma cells respectively. During primary sex differentiation into an ovary after week 8, the primordial germ cells become oogonia and meiosis occurs until birth; in contrast, testicular meiosis begins only at puberty. The neonate carries up to one million ova, which have survived the atresia of most of the 6-7 million that were present at gestational month 6.

Ova proliferate maximally at gestational weeks 16-20; granulosa cells appear at weeks 15-20, interstitial cells at weeks 12-15, and thecal cells during the last trimester.

From birth until puberty, the ovary remains in a resting phase, while extragonadal sexual structures develop. Testicular testosterone and anti-Müllerian hormone are necessary for this secondary sex differentiation in the male, but in the female it occurs in the absence of any positive influences from the ovary; gonadal and genital differentiation are independent phenomena. This is a crucial difference between female and male sexual differentiation.

Table 1 Stages of human ovarian and testicular development

Stage and timing	Morphology and function
1 Pregonadal	
Day 4.5	Primordial germ cells differentiate
2 Indifferent	
Days 7-10	Gonadal ridge differentiates
Up to day 20	Primordial germ cells migrate to gonad primordium on genital ridge
Weeks 5-6	Indifferent gonad formed, with primordial germ cells, coelomic epithelial cells and mesenchymal cells
3 Primary sex differentiation	
Weeks 6-7 to week 8	Male: Sertoli cells and testicular cords develop
	Female: no sign of differentiation
From week 8	Ovarian morphological differentiation
Weeks 9-10	Primordial germ cells develop into oogonia
Weeks 11-12 to neonate	Meiosis begins, up to diplotene of prophase of 1st meiotic division
Neonate-puberty	Resting stage
4 Secondary sex differentiation	
Postnatal week 7-puberty	Male: testicular testosterone and anti-Müllerian hormone produced
	Female: no gonadal factors produced

Studies of Turner's syndrome, in which one X-chromosome is missing, show that both X-chromosomes are needed for meiosis and survival of oogonia. Primordial germ cells migrate to the genital ridge and undergo mitosis normally in Turner's syndrome, but no meiosis occurs, atresia is accelerated, and few or no follicles remain at birth.

Development of follicles

The development of a mammalian ovarian follicle is illustrated in Figure 1. It is a two-stage process. *Folliculogenesis*, with mitosis and early meiosis, occurs in the embryonic and foetal period; the process is gonadotrophin-independent, and requires the presence of two X-chromosomes. *Follicular maturation* continues from foetal into adult life; it occurs at a very low level in early life and is re-activated at puberty. The process becomes gonadotrophin-dependent from the early antral stage onwards; so it appears that gonadotrophin action begins *in utero*.

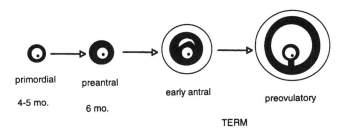

primordial
4-5 mo.

preantral
6 mo.

early antral

preovulatory

TERM

Fig. 1 Stages of mammalian follicular maturation.

Endocrinological development of the ovary

Onset of gonadotrophin action in the developing ovary

Clear-cut direct data on the effects of gonadotrophin on the foetal, neonatal or prepubertal human ovary are lacking; receptor and stimulation tests have not been performed, and most evidence is indirect or comes from studies on animals (1). It seems that luteinizing hormone (LH) and follicle-stimulating hormone (FSH) receptors are absent in the 1st-2nd trimester foetal ovary (2),and that ovarian development is normal in anencephalic foetuses up to week 32 (3), suggesting that gonadotrophins are not necessary for early development. In addition, FSH receptors are found in near-term rhesus monkey ovaries, and ovarian thecal cells, probably with LH receptors, appear during the latter half of gestation (2).

Follicular development to the antral stage, which requires the action of gonadotrophin, occurs near term, suggesting that FSH receptors are present (1). It is likely that prepubertal ovaries have gonadotrophin receptors but that these are not functional in the absence of physiologically significant gonadotrophin secretion.

Very high levels of gonadotrophins in the foetal circulation in the middle of the foetal period decline towards the end of gestation; a likely explanation for the decline is that gonadotrophin secretion is suppressed by the high levels of placental oestrogen. Of the ovarian cells responsive to gonadotrophins, luteal, thecal and interstitial cells respond to LH; granulosa cells respond initially to FSH and later also to LH.

Onset of ovarian steroidogenesis

Even during the first trimester the foetal ovary has all the enzymes needed for steroidogenesis, but for unknown reasons their level of activity is extremely low (1). The interstitial cells are probably the first sites of steroidogenesis, followed by the thecal and granulosa cells, and the gonadotrophin response appears during the third trimester (1, 2). However, at these early stages, the physiological response appears to be minimal or absent.

Gonadotrophin receptor gene mutations

Genetic disturbances of gonadotrophin action

Studies on natural and experimental genetic disturbances of gonadotrophin action in humans and animals have helped to elucidate the early physiology of gonadotrophin action. They include activating and inactivating mutations of the gonadotrophin and gonadotrophin receptor genes in humans, and syndromes including hypogonadotrophic hypogonadism (4-6). In addition, animal data have recently emerged on targeted disruption of gonadotrophin and gonadotrophin receptor genes, producing 'knockout' animals (7, 8), and on natural mutants such as the *hpg* mouse (9), which is hypogonadotrophic due to a deletion in the gonadotrophin-releasing hormone gene. The paper in this volume by Professor Parks also discusses findings on gene mutations and their phenotypes, including hypogonadotrophic hypogonadism e.g. Kallmann's syndrome.

Hypergonadotrophic ovarian dysgenesis (HOD)

HOD is a human disorder in which an inactivating FSH receptor mutation can be involved (10) (although 'dysgenesis' should more properly be 'failure' or 'gonadotrophin resistance'). Table 2 summarizes the characteristics of the syndrome.

Table 2 Characteristics of hypergonadotrophic ovarian 'dysgenesis' (HOD)

Primary or secondary amenorrhoea before 20 years
Normal karyotype (46, XX)
High serum gonadotrophins (FSH>40IU/litre)
No other cause found for the condition
Mendelian recessive inheritance in some cases
Minimum prevalence in Finland 1:8300, carrier frequency 1:45
Inactivating point mutation in FSH receptor gene (Ala 189 Val) causes about 40% of Finnish cases
Mutation frequency lower in other populations

Histologically, the ovaries are full of primordial follicles, with occasional development up to the early preantral stage (11). This picture discriminates HOD patients with the FSH receptor mutation, about 40% of the total in Finland, from those without, in whom no follicles are seen.

Two possible candidate genes were found, one for the LH receptor and one for the FSH receptor. The knowledge that men in affected families who were homozygous for the mutation would be pseudohermaphrodites if the LH receptor were defective (4) showed that the FSH receptor gene is the site of the mutation, because no men were affected in this way (12).

Sequencing the FSH receptor gene from HOD patients revealed a cytosine to thymine mutation in nucleotide 566 in exon 17, such that the amino acid valine (GTA) is expressed instead of alanine (GCA). This small mutation causes a major functional change in the expressed receptor.

With the mutation, very few receptors are expressed at the cell membrane, resulting in only about 3% of the FSH binding found with the normal wild-type receptor, as shown by the cAMP response to FSH stimulation. This finding could explain the phenotype of ovarian failure.

Phenotypes of FSH and LH receptor mutations

One activating FSH receptor mutation (12) and two inactivating mutations have so far been identified (10, 13). In females with HOD, FSH and LH levels are high and secondary sex characters variable; there is primary amenorrhoea and hypoplastic ovaries, and infertility results from arrested follicular maturation (in line with the need for LH for maturation). Males have a normal phenotype with high FSH levels, slightly elevated LH and normal testosterone (14). They have variable reduction of testicular volume and variable spermatogenic suppression, but no azoospermia; on this evidence FSH may not be as important for normal testicular functioning as was thought, which casts doubt on the FSH vaccine approach to male contraception.

Nearly 20 LH receptor mutations have been described, mostly situated in the 6th transmembrane loop of the receptor (6). Activating mutations result in testotoxicosis (male-limited precocious puberty) in males. There is no phenotype in females, because LH has no effect if there has been no previous FSH action; the female with LH alone has no symptoms.

As to inactivating LH receptor mutations, without the action of LH, subjects have a normal female phenotype and ovarian development up to a late stage, but no preovulatory or ovulatory stages (6). Affected women have amenorrhoea and never ovulate.

Postscript

The lessons learnt from studying the effects of gonadotrophin receptor mutations can be summed up in the words of Rabinovici & Jaffe (1):

'During normal fetal and postnatal development of the female child there is no apparent evidence for the need of ovarian function. On the other hand, adequate fetal and prepubertal ovarian development is necessary for normal puberty and reproductive life.'

References

1   Rabinovici J & Jaffe RB. Development and regulation of growth and differentiated function in human and subhuman primate fetal gonads. *Endocrinological Reviews* 1990 **11** 532-557.

2   Huhtaniemi IT, Yamamoto M, Jalkanen J, Ranta T & Jaffe RB. FSH receptors appear earlier in the primate fetal testis than in the ovary. *Journal of Clinical Endocrinology and Metabolism* 1987 **65** 1210-1214.

3   Baker TG & Scrimgeour JB. Development of the gonad in normal and anencephalic human fetuses. *Journal of Reproduction and Fertility* 1980 **60** 193-199.

4   Weiss J, Axelrod L, Whitcomb RW, Harris PE, Crowley WF & Jameson JL. Hypogonadism caused by a single amino acid substitution in the beta subunit of luteinizing hormone. *New England Journal of Medicine* 1992 **326** 179-183.

5   Matthews CH, Borgato S, Beck-Peccoz P, Adams M, Tone Y, Gambino G, Casagrande S, Tedeschini G, Benedetti A & Chatterjee VKK. Primary amenorrhoea and infertility due to a mutation of the beta-subunit of follicle-stimulating hormone. *Nature Genetics* 1993 **5** 83-86.

6   Themmen APN, Martens JWM & Brunner HG. Gonadotropin receptor mutations. *Journal of Endocrinology* 1997 **153** 179-181.

7   Kendall TR, Samuelson LC, Saunders TL, Wood RI & Camper SA. Targeted disruption of the pituitary glycoprotein hormone alpha-subunit produces hypogonadal and hypothyroid mice. *Genes and Development* 1995 **9** 2007-2019.

8   Kumar TR, Wang Y, Lu N & Matzuk MM. Follicle stimulating hormone is required for ovarian follicle maturation but not male fertility. *Nature Genetics* 1997 **15** 201-204.

9   Cattanach BM, Iddon CA, Charlton HM, Chiappa SA & Fink G. Gonadotrophin-releasing hormone deficiency in a mutant mouse with hypogonadism. *Nature* 1977 **269** 338-340.

10   Aittomäki K, Dieguez Lucena JL, Pakarinen P, Sistonen P, Tapanainen J, Gromoll J, Kaskikari R, Sankila E-M, Lehväslaiho H, Reyes Engel A, Nieschlag E, Huhtaniemi I, & de la Chapelle A. Mutation in the follicle-stimulating hormone receptor gene causes hereditary hypergonadotropic ovarian failure. *Cell* 1995 **82** 959-968.

11   Aittomäki K, Herva R, Stenman U-H, Juntunen K, Ylöstalo P, Hovatta O, & de la Chapelle A. Clinical features of primary ovarian failure caused by a point mutation in the follicle-stimulating hormone receptor gene. *Journal of Clinical Endocrinology and Metabolism* 1996 **81** 3722-3726.

12   Gromoll J, Simoni M & Nieschlag E. An activating mutation of the follicle-stimulating hormone receptor autonomously sustains spermatogenesis in a hypophysectomized man. *Journal of Clinical Endocrinology and Metabolism* 1996 **811** 1367-1370.

13   Kotlar TJ, Young RH, Albanese C, Crowley WF Jr, Scully RE & Jameson JL. A mutation in the follicle-stimulating hormone receptor occurs frequently in human ovarian sex cord tumors. *Journal of Clinical Endocrinology and Metabolism* 1997 **82** 1020-1086.

14   Tapanainen JS, Aittomäki K, Juang M, Vaskivuo T & Huhtaniemi IT. Men homozygous for an inactivating mutation of the follicle-stimulating hormone (FSH) receptor gene present variable suppression of spermatogenesis and fertility. *Nature Genetics* 1997 **15** 205-206.

Adolescent Endocrinology
Ed R Stanhope
BioScientifica Ltd, Bristol (1998)

Menarche

M Rees

John Radcliffe Hospital, Oxford, UK

This paper discusses the factors that determine the age of menarche, the process of menstruation and the events in later life that are governed by the age at which menarche occurs. Menarcheal age continues to fall, while age at menopause has long been steady at about 50 years. Thus it is the age at which menarche occurs that determines the duration of a woman's exposure to oestrogen.

Factors affecting age at menarche

Table 1 summarizes some factors affecting age at menarche.

Table 1 Factors determining age at menarche

Genetics
Body weight and composition
Exercise
Season
Family size
Birth order
Chronic illness
Socioeconomic factors

Genetics
There is a greater concordance of age at menarche between identical than between non-identical twins and in mother and daughter pairs than in other populations.

Body weight and composition
Rose Frisch's theory proposes a definite weight:height ratio at which menarche occurs (1), and it is well known that malnourished women have either delayed menarche or secondary amenorrhoea. Frisch described a mean weight and height at menarche of 47.8 kg and 158.5 cm, together with a relative increase in body fat. However this is not now thought to be a key factor.

Recent work from Cyrus Cooper's team in Southampton on the birth cohort of 1946 showed positive relationships between greater birthweight and later menarche, and between greater weight at 7 years and earlier menarche. These observations are consistent with the hypothesis that menarcheal age is linked to programmed patterns of gonadotrophin release, established *in utero* when the fetal hypothalamus is imprinted, and subsequently modified by weight gain in childhood (2).

Exercise

There is concern that women who exercise often can become amenorrhoeic and consequently suffer osteoporosis in later life. In addition, each year of premenarcheal training may be associated with a delay in menarche by 5 months. However, this effect was found in gymnasts but not in tennis players training to the same level (3). It seems that familial and sport-specific factors are involved, so that women who have a late menarche are also those who excel at certain types of sport.

Season

Menarche occurs more frequently in summer and winter, but the reason is not known.

Family size and birth order

Menarche occurs later the larger the family, although children born later in a sibship have an earlier menarche than those born earlier (4).

Chronic illness

Chronic illness such as diabetes or sickle-cell disease will delay menarche.

Decline in menarcheal age over time

In 1840 the mean menarcheal age in Europe was 16 years, but by 1960 it had declined to 13 years. However, this decline has now ceased in some countries, including the UK and Italy, but not in others (5). Reasons for this might be that:

- childhood nutrition and care are now maximal, so that menarcheal age can fall no further
- health and environmental conditions have deteriorated, halting the fall
- girls with later menarche have been genetically selected.

Menstruation

Blood loss

Between the menarche and the menopause a woman in Western society experiences about 400 menstruations, each lasting 5-6 days, a lifetime total of 6-7 years of bleeding. The classic population study of Hallberg *et al.* (6) in Göteborg, Sweden found that menstrual blood loss has a skewed distribution, with a mean of 35 ml/period and a 90th centile value of 80 ml. Blood loss greater than 80 ml constitutes objective menorrhagia, and the highest loss recorded in this study was 540 ml (5). However, a patient in her mid-30s whom my colleagues and I examined in Oxford was losing a world record of 1600 ml/period and described equally heavy periods since her teens.

Duration

My own study of 321 premenopausal women has shown that the average duration of menstruation, experienced by about half of the women, was 5-6 days.

Cycle length

Vollman, in his classic study of nearly 32 000 menstrual cycles in over 650 women aged 11 to 58 years, found that the 'normal' 28 days is only just the most usual cycle length and is experienced by only 13% of women (7). Treloar *et al.* reported similar findings (8). 'Menstrual chaos', with very short or very long cycles, is common in the immediate postmenarcheal phase, because the first few cycles tend to be anovular; only by the 6th postmenarcheal year are even four-fifths of cycles ovular. Ignorance of the great variation in normal physiology on the part of women and their doctors can result in inappropriate management.

The endometrium and menstruation

Only humans and some other primates menstruate; the menstrual cycle involves a series of endometrial events mediated by oestradiol and progesterone, and menstruating species are characterized by spiral arterioles in the endometrium, from which half of menstrual blood is lost. The blood vessels in human endometrium have the unique property of undergoing benign angiogenesis; they grow and regress with each cycle. Angiogenesis is otherwise restricted to malignant disease or wound healing.

Endometrial angiogenesis

Our group has recently been studying models of endometrial angiogenesis. The three basic cell types in the endometrium are the steroid-receptor-positive epithelial and stromal cells, and the vessel endothelial cells, which have no steroid receptors; the hypothesis is as follows.

1 Oestrogen acts not directly on the vessel endothelium, but on the cells of the epithelium or stroma.
2 The epithelium or stroma produces angiogenic regulators.
3 The regulators act on the endothelium.

Stromal cells are relatively easy to culture, but we have been able for the first time to maintain long-lived (months) cultures of non-malignant endometrial epithelial cells; the method involves collagenase digestion, sieving, trypsin/DNase treatment, and resuspension in Dulbecco's modified Eagle's medium/HEPES plus 10% foetal calf serum, with the essential addition of endothelial cell growth supplement (an extract of bovine brain).

The many angiogenic growth factors produced by the cultured epithelial cells include acidic and basic fibroblast growth factor, vascular endothelial growth factor (VEGF), midkine (MK), transforming growth factor β_1, pleotrophin and thymidine phosphorylase. Placental growth factor (related to VEGF) was not found (9).

Effects of steroid hormones

It was found that VEGF and MK were stimulated by oestradiol in epithelial and stromal cells, MK was inhibited by progesterone in epithelial cells, and transforming growth factor β_1 was inhibited by oestrogen and progesterone in epithelial but not in stromal cells; oestrogen and progesterone alone did not significantly affect thymidine phosphorylase expression, but this was markedly upregulated by a combination of progesterone and transforming growth factor β_1.

Endothelial cell culture and angiogenesis

Published claims to have cultured endometrial vessel endothelial cells proved to be mistaken, or the cells quickly died; however, we were able to culture these cells by meeting their very specific growth requirements (e.g. high magnesium and serum concentration, fibronectin- or collagen-coated culture vessels). Growth of the cells was also dependent on VEGF, but epidermal growth factor, basic fibroblast growth factor and interleukin-4 had no effect.

A key role for VEGF in endometrial angiogenesis is suggested by the unique responsiveness of the endothelium to this factor, and by the fact that its expression is regulated by oestradiol and progesterone.

Contraception and termination

At menarche comes fertility, and with it the need for contraception and the risk of teenage pregnancy. The oral contraceptive pill is the method of choice, although a recent 'pill scare' resulting in girls suddenly stopping the pill increased the termination rate in Oxford by 9%, which was also the national trend. Concerns have been expressed that depot contraceptive formulations may diminish bone density, but an ongoing study so far shows no effect on bone (10).

Terminations are either surgical or medical (with mifepristone and prostaglandins). The latter is preferable for young girls if they have parental support.

Pregnancy

Pregnancy itself is not without risks to the mother and the foetus. If the pregnancy is concealed, the mother will have no antenatal care, and may present with pre-eclampsia or preterm labour, which is a common cause of abdominal pain presenting to casualty officers. Often, the pelvis may not be sufficiently developed, resulting in a high risk of operative delivery. In addition, the foetus may suffer from prematurity or intrauterine growth retardation. Pregnancy in the teens is not ideal.

Menarche and disease in later life

Age of menarche can determine the risk of certain diseases in later life.

Non-malignant diseases

Paganini-Hill & Henderson (11) reported an increased risk of Alzheimer's disease in women who had undergone menarche from 14 years onwards, although other studies have not confirmed this. Early menarche can increase the risk of cardiovascular disease, which is the major killer of postmenopausal women in Western societies. In the UK, at least 110 000 women will die from these causes every year. Breast cancer affects 1:12 women in the UK, but comes a long way behind cardiovascular disease in terms of mortality. As to late menarche and bone density, no studies have yet shown a clear difference in frequency of osteoporosis in women who underwent a late menarche; however, a later menarche might mean less bone deposition because of a lower total oestrogen exposure.

Malignant disease

Effects of age at menarche on colorectal, ovarian and renal cancer are still a matter of debate. The effects of various factors in increasing the risks of breast cancer are shown in Table 2. A positive family history, atypical hyperplasia and lobular carcinoma-*in situ* increase the risk most. Early menarche is a relatively minor risk factor (×1.3).

Table 2 Risk factors for breast cancer

Factor	Risk elevation
Early menarche	1.3
Late menopause	1.5
Nulliparity	1.9
Late age at first pregnancy	1.9
Family history of breast cancer	≤4
Proliferative breast disease	1.9
Atypical hyperplasia	4.4
Lobular carcinoma-*in situ*	6.9-12

Menarche and the breast

The lobules of the breast differentiate into different types at various life stages. Type I is undifferentiated, with high proliferation index, and is seen at menarche. Type II appears for a few cycles, to be followed by Types III and

IV, which are highly differentiated, with low proliferation, after pregnancy and lactation. Carriers of the BRCA1 gene do not change from Type I to Type IV, and Type I and Type II lobules can lead to malignant changes such as ductal carcinoma-*in situ* and lobular carcinoma. But Types III and IV give rise only to benign changes such as hyperplasia, cysts and lactating adenomas.

Conclusion

Menarche and the age at which it occurs sets the scene for a series of life events which produces a monthly incapacity for some women, and will continue to govern their lives into their fifth and sixth decades.

References

1 Frisch RE. The right weight: body fat, menarche and ovulation. *Baillère's Clinical Obstetrics and Gynecology* 1990 **4** 419-439.

2 Cooper C, Kuh D, Egger P, Wadsworth M & Barker D. Childhood growth and age at menarche. *British Journal of Obstetrics and Gynaecology* 1996 **103** 814-817.

3 Malina RM, Ryan RC & Bonci CM. Age at menarche in athletes and their mothers and sisters. *Annals of Human Biology* 1994 **21** 417-422.

4 Roberts DF, Rotner LM, & Swan AV. Age at menarche, physique and environment in industrial north east England. *Acta Paediatrica Scandinavica* 1971 **60** 158-164.

5 Baxter-Jones ADG, Helms P, Baines-Preece J & Preece M. Menarche in intensively trained gymnasts, swimmers and tennis players. *Annals of Human Biology* 1994 **21** 407-415.

6 Hallberg L, Hogdahl AM, Nilsson I & Rybo G. Menstrual blood loss: a population study. *Acta Obstetrica et Gynecologica Scandinavica* 1966 **45** 320-351.

7 Vollman RF. *The Menstrual Cycle*. Philadelphia: Saunders 1977.

8 Treloar AE, Boynton RE, Behn BG & Brown BW. Variation of the human menstrual cycle throughout reproductive life. *International Journal of Fertility* 1967 **12** 77-126.

9 Zhang L, Rees MCP & Bicknell R. The isolation and long-term culture of normal human endometrial endothelium and stroma: expression of mRNAs for angiogenic polypeptides basally and on oestrogen and progesterone challenges. *Journal of Cell Science* 1995 **108** 323-331.

10 Grimwood J, Bicknell R & Rees MCP. The isolation, characterization and culture of human decidual endothelium. *Human Reproduction* 1995 **8** 2142-2148.

11 Paganini-Hill A & Henderson VW 1994. Estrogen deficiency and risk of Alzheimer's disease in women. *American Journal of Epidemiology* 1994 **140** 256-261.

Gonadotrophic requirements for ovulation in adolescent girls

D Baird

Department of Obstetrics and Gynaecology, Centre for
Reproductive Biology, University of Edinburgh, Edinburgh, UK

This paper first takes adolescence as a model system for considering the gonadotrophin requirements for the induction of ovulation, and goes on to report on some studies in which recombinant gonadotrophins have been used for the first time in attempts to simulate the physiological requirements for induction. In future, long-acting combined follicle-stimulating hormone (FSH) and human chorionic gonadotrophin could be used to induce puberty and spermatogenesis in males. A short-acting agonist would allow more accurate treatment. Gonadotrophin antagonists are also in development.

Adolescence: requirements for ovulation

FSH and luteinizing hormone (LH)

As Professor Huhtaniemi explains elsewhere in this volume, follicles grow throughout life from the foetal stage to the menopause (by which time the stock of oocytes is exhausted). For the first 4-5 months, follicle development does not need gonadotrophin, and only at a late stage, when the antral follicle is about 2 mm in diameter, does it require exposure to a coordinated sequence of gonadotrophins for ovulation to occur.

The developing antral follicle first requires FSH; this appears to induce a series of crucial changes in the maturation and differentiation of the granulosa cells which lead to the preovulatory follicle stage. Changes in the expression of gonadotrophin receptors throughout this period include particularly the acquisition by the granulosa cells of LH receptors, which hitherto have been confined to the thecal layer. The follicle can now respond to the preovulatory surge of LH which is essential for ovulation, and for the granulosa cells to form the corpus luteum.

The granulosa cells of the mature Graafian follicle still have FSH receptors, but the unique ability of the mature follicle to sustain its terminal growth and differentiation by way of LH distinguishes it from earlier antral follicles which depend solely on FSH.

Gonadotrophin-releasing hormone (GnRH)

In order for levels of FSH to exceed the threshold necessary to induce the maturational changes in the granulosa cells allowing them to respond to LH, the hypothalamic/pituitary unit must be able to generate a pulsatile secretion of GnRH at a minimum frequency of one per hour. The ovary can function and produce oestrogen-secreting follicles with a lower GnRH pulse rate; but ovulation does not then occur, because the pituitary must be primed at a rate of at least one per hour for a few days before it can respond to oestrogen with an ovulatory surge of LH.

The ovarian cycle and ovarian failure

Ovarian cycle patterns

Ovarian cycle patterns in adolescent girls range from 'normal', through cycles with an inadequate luteal phase, short follicular phase or long follicular phase (1), to anovulatory cycles. These patterns probably reflect the relative immaturity of the hypothalamic/pituitary unit rather than any defect in folliculogenesis. Different cycle patterns have been described in the gynaecological literature for over a century.

Ovulatory failure

Many years ago my colleagues and I in Edinburgh investigated the endocrine background of ovulatory failure in a girl who underwent menarche at 12 and subsequently suffered irregular bleeding associated with fluctuating urinary secretion. She had no ovulation, despite very high oestrogen peaks which would normally provoke a positive feedback response (2). Five years later we challenged a group of such adolescent girls whose presenting symptom was irregular bleeding with exogenous oestrogen (e.g. ethinyloestradiol, 200 µg/ day for 3 days). In contrast with normal women, they showed an absent or impaired LH response to the oestrogen stimulus. The defect causing this is not understood, but probably acts at anterior pituitary level (3). Evidently the hypothalamic/pituitary/ovarian axis must be intact for a coordinated release of gonadotrophins during the follicular phase.

Inhibin

Our knowledge of the feedback mechanism has been enhanced by the recent discovery of the glycoprotein hormone inhibin, which is produced by the granulosa cells of the follicle and contributes to the feedback effect at the level of the anterior pituitary by suppressing levels of FSH. Circulating oestradiol is produced largely from the dominant follicle, and this is presumably the main signal from the ovary to the central nervous system. By contrast, inhibin derives not only from the dominant follicle, but also from the smaller antral follicles. So oestradiol and inhibin probably give somewhat different information to the hypothalamic/pituitary unit even though they can both suppress FSH.

A further complication is that inhibin is dimeric, and that the patterns of secretion of inhibin A and B differ at different stages of the cycle. Inhibin A secretory patterns closely resemble those of oestradiol, rising to a peak in the luteal phase, whereas inhibin B peaks early, declining from the mid-follicular phase, peaking briefly again around ovulation, and declining considerably during the luteal phase. The current hypothesis is that inhibin B arises from the smaller antral follicles, at about the time that they are stimulated by FSH, whereas inhibin A is produced by the dominant follicle and the corpus luteum.

Mechanism of selection of a dominant follicle

The changes in the concentrations of inhibin A and B reflect the development of the pool of antral follicles from which one will become dominant. The selection mechanism is not fully understood, but the intercycle increase in FSH level probably allows the largest available non-atretic small follicle to be activated, and to become dominant by suppressing FSH level below that needed to mediate maturation. Probably oestradiol and possibly inhibin A play a signalling role in this process.

Induction of ovulation

How can the physiological principles of the normal cycle be applied to the induction of ovulation in anovulatory women? Over 30 years ago Gemzell first described induction of ovulation in anovulatory women, using extracts of human pituitary gonadotrophin (4), and later Lunenfeld and colleagues used urinary extracts of FSH and LH (5). Preparations used at this time contained less than 5% gonadotrophins, but by the mid 1980s advances in chromatography enabled FSH preparations of more than 98% (e.g. Metrodin HP) to be prepared, and more recently recombinant FSH and LH of greater than 99% purity have become available.

Potential of new recombinant gonadotrophins

Advantages of recombinant preparations

These new preparations are purer than the extracts previously available, their quality is more reproducible, they can be administered by subcutaneous injection (including self-administration) because they contain little protein contamination, and they are more reliably available than urinary extracts.

Clinical applications of recombinant gonadotrophins

The dominant worldwide use of FSH, the stimulation of multiple follicular development of *in vitro* fertilization (IVF) and embryo transfer, has contributed to the current shortage of gonadotrophins. However, induction of ovulation could be considered a more rewarding application, because its therapeutic aim is to produce a single ovulation, with a low incidence of hyperstimulation and consequent multiple pregnancy.

Induction of ovulation

The two main indications for ovulatory induction are:
- hypogonadotrophic hypogonadism (e.g. Kallman's syndrome)
- normogonadotrophic anovulation (polycystic ovary; PCO).

The effective safe replacement therapy of choice in nearly all women with hypogonadotrophic hypogonadism is pulsatile GnRH, because their anterior pituitary is intact, and only GnRH secretion is deficient. Similarly, most women with PCO can be successfully treated with antioestrogens, but gonadotrophins are to be considered in hypopituitary women, those who lack a pituitary, and those who fail to ovulate in response to antioestrogens.

Hypogonadotrophic hypogonadism Schoot *et al.* (6) first showed (in a woman with Kallman's syndrome) that recombinant FSH could successfully induce follicular development. This single case showed that it was possible to induce the development of large antral follicles within 2 weeks, even though the patient had received little gonadotrophin, and that follicle development can be induced with FSH alone, without LH, although, without LH, oestrogen is not secreted and the end organ (the endometrium) is not stimulated.

A trial was conducted by Serono Laboratories in which hypogonadotrophic women received recombinant FSH, 150 IU/day together with LH, 0, 25, 75 or 225 IU. Only those women receiving the two highest doses of LH developed sufficient oestrogen stimulation for ovulation.

Table 1 Results of low-dose gonadotrophin therapy in 100 women with polycystic ovary syndrome (8)

Parameter	Number
Cycles	
Total	401
Ovulatory	289 (72)
Uniovulatory	219 (55)
Pregnancies/outcomes	
Total	45
Abortions + ectopic	19
Multiple	2
Viable births	26 (6.5)

Percentage of total cycles is given in parentheses

Normogonadotrophic anovulation Patients who fail to respond to antioestrogens may need gonadotrophins. Conventional 'step-up' treatment of PCO with gonadotrophins typically results in a high proportion of ovulatory cycles and a reasonable number of pregnancies; but about one quarter of pregnancies are multiple, and 17% miscarry. Consequently, many gonadotrophin dose regimens attempt to duplicate the natural state as accurately as possible. Of these, ultra-low-dose FSH is probably the treatment of choice (7). Its rationale is to top up endogenous FSH to a level at which a follicle is stimulated to develop. Table 1 summarizes a study by Hamilton-Fairley *et al.* (8) in which only two of 45 pregnancies were multiple, but the 'take-home baby rate' was also low, only 6.5%.

Conclusions

Current conclusions as to the requirements for exogenous gonadotrophins are as follows.

- In normogonadotrophic anovulation and for IVF, only FSH is needed because endogenous LH is adequate.
- For hypogonadotrophic women treated with gonadotrophins, LH must be given in addition to FSH, to secure normal oestradiol levels.
- The optimum doses and dose ratios of FSH and LH to achieve mono-ovulation have not yet been established.

The future

Recombinant gonadotrophin technology has not yet been fully exploited. Table 2 summarizes some possible future developments. A long-acting combined FSH and human chorionic gonadotrophin could be particularly useful for inducing puberty and spermatogenesis in males. A short-acting agonist would allow more precise manipulation of the gonadotrophic environment. Gonadotrophic antagonists are in development, and single-chain (rather than dimeric) molecules, retain their biological properties while making available antigenic sites hidden in the tertiary structure of the native molecule.

Table 2 Future developments in gonadotrophin replacement therapy

Long-acting gonadotrophin analogues
e.g. FSHβ - hCG C-terminal extension hybrids
Short-acting agonists
e.g. by diminished glycosylation
Antagonists
site-directed mutagensis; e.g. removal of α52 and β13
Asn N-linked oligosaccharides
Tethered single-chain gonadtrophins

FSH, follicle-stimulating hormone; hCG, human chorionic gonadotrophin

References

1   Apter D, Viinika L & Vihko R. Hormonal pattern of adolescent menstrual cycles. *Journal of Clinical Endocrinology and Metabolism* 1978 **47** 944-945.

2   Fraser IS, Michie IE, Wide L & Baird DT. Pituitary gonadotrophins and ovarian function in adolescent dysfunctional uterine bleeding. *Journal of Clinical Endocrinology and Metabolism* 1973 **37** 407-412.

3   Van Look PFA, Hunter WM, Fraser IS & Baird DT. Impaired estrogen-induced luteinizing hormone release in adolescents with anovulatory dysfunctional uterine bleeding. *Journal of Clinical Endocrinology and Metabolism* 1978 **46** 816-823.

4   Gemzell CA, Diczfalusy E & Tillinger G. Clinical effect of human pituitary follicle-stimulating hormone (FSH). *Journal of Clinical Endocrinology and Metabolism* 1958 **18** 1333-1348.

5   Lunenfeld B & Insler V. Induction of ovulation: historical aspects. *Ballière's Clinics in Obstetrics and Gynaecology* 1990 **4** 473-490.

6   Schoot DC, Coelingh Bennink HJT, Mannaerts BMJL, Lamberts SWJ, Bouchard P & Fauser BCJM. Human recombinant follicle-stimulating hormone induces growth of preovulatory follicles without concomitant increase in androgen and estrogen biosynthesis in a woman with isolated gonadotropin deficiency. *Journal of Clinical Endocrinology and Metabolism* 1992 **74** 1471-1473.

7   White DM, Polson DW, Kiddy, Sagle P, Watson H, Gilling-Smith C, Hamilton-Fairley D & Franks S. Induction of ovulation with low dose gonadotropins in polycystic ovary syndrome: an analysis of 109 pregnancies in 225 women. *Journal of Clinical Endocrinology and Metabolism* 1996 **81** 3821-3824.

8   Hamilton-Fairley D, Kiddy D, Watson H, Sagle M & Franks S. Low-dose gonadotrophin therapy for induction of ovulation in 100 women with polycystic ovary syndrome. *Human Reproduction* 1991 **6** 1095-1099.

Adolescent Endocrinology
Ed R Stanhope
BioScientifica Ltd, Bristol (1998)

Outlook for males with hypogonadotrophic hypogonadism

M Vandeweghe

Department of Endocrinology, University Hospital, Ghent, Belgium

Hypogonadotrophic hypogonadism (HH) in males is a hypothalamo-pituitary disorder in which either the hypothalamic pulsatile luteinizing hormone-releasing hormone (LHRH) secretion is definitely absent or the pituitary cannot produce enough luteinizing hormone and follicle-stimulating hormone. Both result in deficient testosterone production and spermatogenesis. This condition should be distinguished, often with difficulty in clinical practice, from extreme delay in puberty, in which subjects eventually achieve complete virilization.

This chapter is concerned almost exclusively with males who suffer from permanent HH that is already present before the completion of pubertal development, and I will deal only briefly with patients with definite HH, acquired in adulthood after complete virilization and fertility has been obtained via normal adolescence. In these males, in which gonadotrophic deficiency develops as the result of a pituitary tumour for instance, a short course of gonadotrophin treatment (even sometimes human choriogonadotrophin (hCG) alone) is generally effective in restoring fertility, if required, and testosterone substitution will solve the problems of the associated androgen deficiency.

The causes of prepubertal HH include congenital defects, tumours, pituitary trauma and radiotherapy (see Table 1). They can lead to either isolated HH or HH associated with deficiencies of other hormones. The therapeutic approach to, and outlook for, these two patient groups are discussed separately.

Table 1 Major aetiologies of prepubertal hypogonadotrophic hyogonadism

---

Congenital
  Development defects of the central nervous system (e.g. Kallmann's
  syndrome, septo-optic dysplasia)
  Traumatic (breech) delivery
Tumours (e.g. craniopharyngioma)
Post-traumatic (e.g. stalk section)
Post-radiotheraphy (e.g. haematological malignancy)
Other causes (rare)

Treatment of patients with combined growth hormone and gonadotrophic deficiency

Children with such disorders have combined growth hormone and gonadotrophin deficiency often associated with deficiencies of thyroid stimulating hormone and adrenocorticotrophic hormone.

Delaying testosterone replacement therapy?

Important work on the management of such children, particularly the induction of puberty, was published in 1986 by the Belgian Study Group for Paediatric Endocrinology (1). The study demonstrated a significant negative linear relationship between bone age velocity during puberty and bone age at onset of puberty. Mean bone age increment per chronological year was over 1.5 years when puberty started at a bone age of 11 years, but only half that value when puberty was induced at a bone age of 15 years. Delaying the onset of testosterone replacement therapy in these hypopituitary boys results in greater stature at the start of puberty, combined with a smaller than normal subsequent loss in height incremental gain, producing an actually improved final height (about 5 cm with therapy onset at a bone age of 15 years).

These theoretical benefits of late onset of androgen therapy are clinically irrelevant, however, when the severe psychosexual problems caused by late pubertal induction are taken into account. Therefore the actual therapeutic policy in this patient population, after optimized long-term growth hormone therapy, consists of pubertal induction with increasing doses of testosterone (50-200 mg/month), starting at a chronological age of 14-16 years, while continuing growth hormone treatment.

This approach results in young adults with optimal growth spurt and virilization, but whose testes have not yet developed beyond the prepubertal stage. For such patients, textbooks of paediatric endocrinology recommend postponing treatment with gonadotrophins or LHRH 'until fertility is asked for', because 'their efficiency is not reduced by previous testosterone treatment' (2, 3).

Reasons for not delaying fertility induction

We feel that there are two good reasons for not delaying induction of fertility in these patients. First it has not been definitely established that the hypothalamo-pituitary-testicular axis will react adequately after years of inactivity during testosterone substitution, so that fertility is fully restored (4). Secondly, most patients do not return later to 'ask for fertility'. The reasons for this are that they are psychologically distressed and refrain from embarking on a relationship because they are incompletely virilized, have an empty scrotum and entertain severe doubts about their ultimate fertility.

Poor psychosexual adjustment

Data from France, Canada, the USA and elsewhere clearly show that the social and psychosexual adjustment of such hypopituitary patients (particularly males) is very poor when they reach adulthood. Consequently the proportion of married subjects is particularly low compared with unaffected controls. Dean *et al.* (5) in Canada showed that only about 15% of 116 hypopituitary patients (with either isolated HH or multiple hormone deficiency) were in a stable relationship, compared with nearly 70% of a matched control population. Of 21 patients over 25 years of age with growth hormone deficiency and HH, only 4 (19%) were married or had a stable relationship, compared with 10 of 24 (42%) with growth hormone deficiency but no associated hypogonadism. Job *et al.* (6) in France found a similarly low proportion of married males in the hypopituitary adult population.

The possible reasons for social and psychosexual maladjustment are shown in Table 2.

Table 2 Reasons for social-sexual maladjustment in hypopituitary males

1. Growth retardation →short adult stature
2. Delay in pubertal development
3. Incomplete puberty
   'Weak' male phenotype (beard, pubic and axillary hair)
   Small prepubertal testes ('empty scrotum')
4. Questionable fertility
5. Growth hormone-deficient adult (bone, muscle, general well-being)

Gonadotrophin therapy for hypopituitary males

In order to achieve near-normal testicular development, improve the chances of fertility and thus provide psychological benefit, we systematically use gonadotrophin therapy after primary virilization with testosterone. The first therapeutic results were published several years ago (7). hCG, 1500U, was given once a week for 3 months, and human menopausal gonadotrophin (hMG), 150U 2 or 3 times a week, was then added for 12-18 months.

With this regimen, testicular volume was below 3 ml in all patients before treatment, and with hMG treatment increased progressively up to a mean of 15 ml. In 12 of 16 patients (in which a testicular volume of more than 12 ml was obtained) sperm density was 10 million or more per ml.

Thus treatment with combined gonadotrophins for 12-18 months produced an adult testicular volume and a satisfactory sperm density in most hypopituitary males with combined growth hormone and gonadotrophin deficiency. It is evident that this approach, in completing the male phenotype of the patient, will confer substantial psychological benefits. As Quinton and Bouloux (4) point out, it is worth giving such male patients replacement therapy with hCG/hMG or pulsatile LHRH when they reach 18-20 years, even if fertility is not immediately needed. The reason for this is that earlier stimulation probably leads to better spermatogenesis with subsequent stimulation and that patients are also very grateful for the increase in testicular volume.

Treatment of patients with isolated HH

In a few patients with partial HH (initial testicular volume 4 ml), treatment with hCG alone can be effective (8-10), while in the complete form (in which the testicular volume remains prepubertal) the therapeutic options are hCG/hMG or pulsatile LHRH.

Treatment of isolated HH with gonadotrophins

The goals of gonadotrophin treatment are an adult testicular volume, normal spermatogenesis and, ultimately, fertility. Results of studies differ: Nieschlag (11) reported an 80-90% success rate, while Finkel *et al.* (12) found only 40%. It seems likely that most of Finkel's failures were due to pre-existing bilateral cryptorchidism, as I found in my own study of 18 young adult patients with complete isolated HH (unpublished data). Five of my 18 patients had Kallmann's syndrome with anosmia, and eight had a history of surgery for bilateral cryptorchidism. Combined hCG/hMG resulted in success in six patients, with testicular volume rising to 10-18 ml, sperm counts of 2-36 million per ml and pregnancy in the partners of the three subjects who desired it. Little or no beneficial change occurred in 12 patients, including all eight with bilateral cryptorchidism.

Treatment of isolated HH with pulsatile LHRH

In 10 well documented studies (13-22) a total of 149 patients received pulsatile LHRH, in the majority subcutaneously, by syringe pump, for 6-36 months resulting in consistent increases in testicular volume in 105/110 patients and spermatogenesis in 105/140. Delemarre-Van De Waal (22) reported 'encouraging results' in a series of 28 patients, with a final testicular volume of 10 ml or more in 22 of the 28 patients and acceptable spermatogenesis in 19 of 26 patients. Treatment, however, had to be continued over a long period (about 18 months on average, with a range of 9-36 months).

GnRH versus hCG/hMG treatment in isolated HH

Liu *et al.* (18,23) reported no clear advantage of GnRH over hCG/hMG, but the two treatment groups were not fully comparable. On the other hand, Schopohl *et al.* (21) found GnRH to be superior to hCG/hMG, with a more pronounced increase in testicular volume, quicker onset of spermatogenesis and fewer side effects (e.g. gynecomastia). In addition, other studies have reported successful treatment of isolated HH with GnRH after hCG/hMG had failed, but the total number of patients was rather small (17, 22, 24, 25).

Conclusions

A short course of treatment with gonadotrophins, often hCG alone, effectively restores fertility in the majority of patients with HH acquired in adulthood; the same is true for a subpopulation of patients with partial HH of prepubertal onset.

As to the treatment of male adolescents with prepubertal HH associated with other pituitary hormonal deficiencies (particularly growth hormone), after primary induction of puberty with increasing doses of testosterone, treatment with hCG/hMG or pulsatile LHRH is needed to achieve satisfactory testicular volume and fertility potential.

In patients with isolated HH, treatment with hCG/hMG or pulsatile LHRH will ultimately achieve fertility in one-half to two-thirds of the subjects.

References

1   Bourguignon JP, Vandeweghe M, Vanderschueren-Lodeweyckx M, Malvaux P, Wolter R, Ducaju M & Ernould C. Pubertal growth and final height in hypopituitarism: a minor role of bone age at onset of puberty. *Journal of Clinical Endocrinology and Metabolism* 1986 **63** 376-382.

2   Job JC. Hypogonadism at adolescence: lack or delay of sexual development? In: *Pediatric Endocrinology*, pp 259-266. Ed F Lifshitz. New York: Marcel Dekker, 1996.

3   Bridges NA & Brook CGD. Disorders of puberty. In: *Clinical Paediatric Endocrinology*, pp 253-273. Ed CGD Brook. London: Blackwell Science, 1995.

4   Quinton R & Bouloux PMG. Male hypogonadism, infertility and impotence. In: *Drug Therapy in Reproductive Endocrinology*, pp 242-258. Ed J Ginsburg. London: Arnold, 1996.

5   Dean HJ, Mctaggart TL, Fisk DG & Friesen HG. The educational, vocational and marital status of growth hormone deficient adults, treated with growth hormone during childhood. *American Journal of Diseases of Children* 1985 **139** 1105-1110.

6   Job JC, Chicaud J, Toublanc JE, Chaussain JL, Garnier P, Vassal J *et al.* Le devenir à long terme des nains hypophysaires traités par l'hormone de croissance. *Archives Françaises de Pédiatrie* 1988 **45** 169-173.

7   Vandeweghe M. Complete virilization and spermatogenesis with combined hCG/hMG treatment in gonadotropin and growth hormone deficient patients. In: *Hormonal Regulation of Growth*, pp 283-287. Eds H Frisch H & MO Thorner. New York: Raven Press, 1989.

8   Burris AS, Robard HW, Winters SJ & Sherins RJ. Gonadotropin therapy in men with isolated hypogonadotropic hypogonadism: the response to human chorionic gonadotropin is predicted by initial testicular size. *Journal of Clinical Endocrinology and Metabolism* 1988 **66** 1144-1151.

9   Vicari E, Mongioi A, Calogero AE, Moncada ML, Sidoti G, Polosa P & D'Agata R. Therapy with human chorionic gonadotrophin alone induces spermatogenesis in men with isolated hypogonadotrophic hypogonadism: long-term follow-up. *International Journal of Andrology* 1992 **15** 320-329.

10 Kung AWC, Zhong YY, Lam KSL & Wang C. Induction of spermatogenesis with gonadotrophins in Chinese men with hypogonadotrophic hypogonadism. *International Journal of Andrology* 1994 **17** 241-247.

11   Nieschlag E. Development of spermatogenesis. Lecture given at the 35th Annual Meeting of the European Society for Paediatric Endocrinology (ESPE) Montpellier France 15-18 September 1996.

12   Finkel DM, Phillips JL & Snyder PJ. Stimulation of spermatogenesis by gonadotropins in men with hypogonadotropic hypogonadism. *New England Journal of Medicine* 1985 **313** 651-655.

13   Hoffman AR & Crowley WF Jr. Induction of puberty in men by long-term pulsatile administration of low-dose gonadotropin releasing hormone. *New England Journal of Medicine* 1982 **307** 1237-1241.

14   Klingmuller D & Schweikert HU. Maintenance of spermatogenesis by intranasal administration of gonadotropin releasing hormone in patients with hypothalamic hypogonadism. *Journal of Clinical Endocrinology and Metabolism* 1985 **61** 868-872.

15   Spratt DI, Finkelstein JS, O'Dea LS, Badger TM, Rao PN, Campbell JD & Crowley WF Jr. Long-term administration of gonadotrophic-releasing hormone in men with idiopathic hypogonadotropic hypogonadism. *Annals of Internal Medicine* 1986 **105** 848-855.

16   Shargil AA. Treatment of idiopathic hypogonadotropic hypogonadism in men with luteinizing hormone-releasing hormone: a comparison of treatment with daily injections and with the pulsatile infusion pump. *Fertility and Sterility* 1987 **47** 492-500.

17   Blumenfeld Z, Frisch L & Conn PM. Gonadotropin releasing hormone (GnRH) antibodies formation in hypogonadotropic azoospermic men treated with pulsatile GnRH: diagnosis and possible alternative treatment. *Fertility and Sterility* 1988 **50** 622-629.

18   Liu L, Banks SM, Barnes KM & Sherins RJ. Two year comparison of testicular responses to pulsatile gonadotropin releasing hormone and exogenous gonadotropins from the inception of therapy in men with isolated hypogonadotropic hypogonadism. *Journal of Clinical Endocrinology and Metabolism* 1988 **67** 1140-1145.

19   Aulitzky W, Frick J & Galvan G. Pulsatile luteinizing hormone-releasing hormone treatment of male hypogonadotropic hypogonadism. *Fertility and Sterility* 1988 **50** 480-486.

20   Whitcomb RW & Crowley WF. Diagnosis and treatment of isolated gonadotropin-releasing hormone deficiency in men. *Journal of Clinical Endocrinology and Metabolism* 1990 **70** 3-7.

21   Schopohl J, Mehltretter G, Von Zumbusch R, Eversmann T & Von Werder K. Comparison of gonadotropin-releasing hormone and gonadotropin therapy in male patients with idiopathic hypothalamic hypogonadism. *Fertility and Sterility* 1991 **56** 1143-1150.

22   Delemarre-Van de Waal HA. Induction of testicular growth and spermatogenesis by pulsatile intravenous administration of gonadotropin-releasing hormone in patients with hypogonadotrophic hypogonadism. *Clinical Endocrinology* 1993 **38** 473-480.

23   Liu L, Chaudhari N, Corle D & Sherins RJ. Comparison of pulsatile subcutaneous gonadotropin-releasing hormone and exogenous gonadotropins in the treatment of men with isolated hypogonadotropic hypogonadism. *Fertility and Sterility* 1988 **49** 302-308.

24   Morris DV, Adeniyi-Jones R, Wheeler M, Sonksen P & Jacobs HS. The treatment of hypogonadrophic hypogonadism in men by the pulsatile infusion of luteinizing hormone releasing hormone. *Clinical Endocrinology* 1984 **21** 189-200.

25   Berezin M, Weissenberg R, Rabinovitch O & Lunenfeld B. Succesful GnRH treatment in a patient with Kallmann's syndrome, who previously failed on hMG/ hCG treatment. *Andrologia* 1988 **20** 285-288.

Adolescent Endocrinology
Ed R Stanhope
BioScientifica Ltd, Bristol (1998)

Management of infertility and the newer reproductive techniques: treatment opportunities and ethical implications

M C Davies

Reproductive Medicine Unit, University College London Hospitals, Huntley Street, London WC1E 6AU, UK

This chapter addresses aspects of endocrine disorders that affect fertility, and presents a general overview of current fertility treatment. It attempts to indicate opportunities that may be available to many adolescents with disorders discussed elsewhere in this publication as they grow into adulthood in the 21st century, opportunities that nevertheless are leading clinicians into a minefield of ethical dilemmas.

Approaches to anovulatory infertility

One notable success story is the treatment of anovulatory infertility. In particular, after 6 months of treatment, women with hypogonadotrophic hypogonadism and amenorrhoea have a virtually normal cumulative conception rate of 80% (Fig. 1) (1). Even women with oligomenorrhoea, most of whom suffer from polycystic ovary syndrome (PCOS), do very well with appropriate treatment.

Treatment with pulsatile gonadotrophin-releasing hormone

The modern syringe pump is elegant both in design and use, and can be a marvellously simple and effective mode of treatment. In a typical case, illustrated in Figure 2, a woman with hypogonadotrophic hypogonadism wore a pump for 2 weeks and received a 15 µg pulse of luteinizing hormone (LH)-releasing hormone (LHRH) every 90 min. A spontaneous LH surge ensued and a corpus luteum was demonstrated on ultrasound scan.

PCOS

Women with anovulatory infertility due to PCOS are more difficult to treat. Treatment begins with weight loss, and 60-70% of such women respond to antioestrogen therapy. Gonadotrophin treatment and laparoscopic ovarian diathermy are therapeutic alternatives.

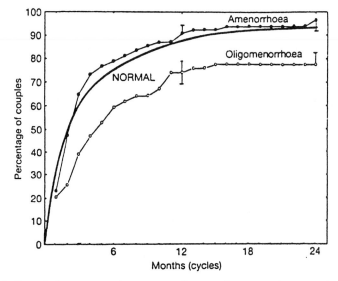

Fig. 1 Cumulative conception rates of anovulatory patients undergoing treatment. Reproduced by permission from (1) © BMJ Publishing Group

Complications of gonadotrophin treatment for anovulatory infertility in the patient with PCOS

Complications of such treatment are threefold. First, there is a risk of multiple birth. The number of triplet and higher-order births has greatly increased in England and Wales over the last 20 years, although, with the legal restriction of the number of embryos replaced in *in vitro* fertilization (IVF) cycles to three, the higher-order multiple births (Fig. 3) (2) are entirely due to *in vivo* induction of ovulation. They give rise to problems of prematurity and handicap.

Ovarian hyperstimulation syndrome (OHSS) is the second complication faced by the patient with PCOS receiving gonadotrophins. Severe OHSS is reported to occur in about 1% of cycles in treated women. Full-blown OHSS presents as massively enlarged ovaries, ascites, pleural effusions and renal impairment (due partly to prerenal dehydration and partly to raised intra-abdominal pressure). OHSS can be a very frightening condition and thromboembolism due to dehydration can be fatal. However, of 800 *in vivo* and *in vitro* gonadotrophin cycles in our unit in 1995, only six patients had to be admitted, although three of these required intensive care. OHSS can be minimized in several ways; if monitoring suggests that a patient is at risk during *in vivo* induction of ovulation the cycle should be abandoned.

The third complication is controversial, but important for practitioners and patients to be aware of; it has long been known that infertile women are at increased risk of ovarian cancer, but infertility drug treatment is associated with further increase in risk. Rossing *et al.* (3) showed that, in a population of

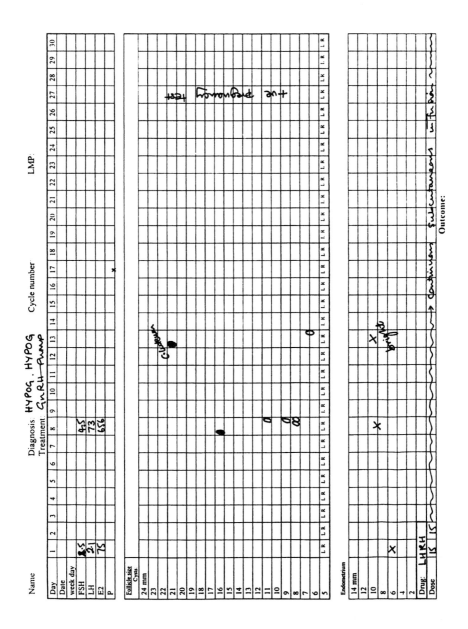

Fig. 2 Ovulation induction treatment cycle using subcutaneous LHRH. Hypog hypog, hypogonadotrophic hypogonadism. GnRH, gonadotrophin releasing hormone. c. luteum, corpus luteum. LR, left and right ovary.

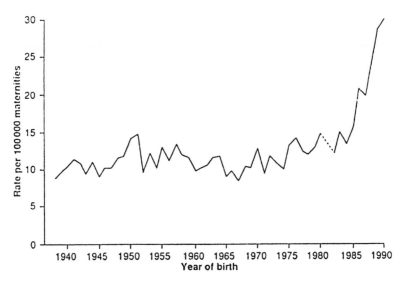

Fig. 3 Proportion of all maternities resulting in a triplet or higher order birth in England and Wales 1939-1990. Reproduced with permission from (2) © Springer-Verlag.

infertile women, those who had not been treated had a relative risk of 1.4, while with long-term clomiphene citrate treatment the relative risk was 3.1, and with gonadotrophins, 5.6. There are concerns that women receiving IVF treatment may also be at increased risk of ovarian tumours.

Laparoscopic ovarian diathermy (LOD)

This technique is being used in PCOS as an alternative to gonadotrophin treatment with its attendant problems, particularly in the slim patient with tonically high LH. Electrodiathermy or a laser is used to drill several defects through the ovarian capsule. Donesky & Adashi (4) reviewed the results of many studies published over the last decade; of 947 women treated with LOD, 82% achieved ovulation and 59% became pregnant. The mechanism of the response to LOD is unknown. The risks of the procedure are surgical, and there is a small chance of adhesion formation. The advantages are that ovulation is unifollicular, cycle monitoring is not necessary, and the miscarriage rate may be reduced.

Congenital adrenal hyperplasia (CAH)

Although males with reduced spermatogenesis due to CAH are said to respond to steroid replacement therapy, women with the disorder have a very low fertility rate. Women with late-onset CAH do better than those with the classical form, although they may require ovulation induction and may have difficulties related to elevated baseline levels of progesterone. Many women with classical

CAH, particularly those with the salt-losing form, face great sexual and marital difficulties (5). Among 15 salt losers, 83% had never married (compared with 10% of the general population), the introitus was inadequate in 53%, 60% had no sexual experience and only 1/15 achieved pregnancy (6). The problems were generally not so severe in non-salt-losers, although only 55% of these had 'normal' menses, compared with 87% of the general population, and 15/25 non-salt-losers became pregnant (6). They may need Caesarean sections because of their short stature. The outlook for women with classical CAH is probably improving as treatment efficacy increases.

Male infertility

Suboptimal semen parameters are identified as the cause of infertility in a quarter of couples presenting for investigation, and there is evidence that average semen quality has declined over the last 40 years. Hypogonadal males can be treated with the LHRH pump or gonadotrophin injections to induce spermatogenesis.

Viable sperm can be concentrated by centrifugation and used for intrauterine insemination, usually in conjunction with superovulation in the woman. With very low counts and/or low motility, IVF is preferred. The outcome of IVF is a 20-25% pregnancy rate, once fertilization and embryo transfer have been achieved. This yields a cumulative conception rate of around 60% after four cycles. Unfortunately in Britain most couples will undertake only one or two cycles of treatment, because of the emotional strain and financial burden. Only one in seven cycles in the UK is currently paid for by the NHS.

Intracytoplasmic sperm injection (ICSI)

With motile sperm counts of one million or less, IVF is likely to fail. Of several micromanipulation techniques developed to help the sperm penetrate the capsule of the zona pellucida and reach the egg, ICSI is the most effective, and its results are extremely good. Of a total of over 10 000 treatment cycles documented in the European Society for Human Reproduction and Embryology registry by 1994, a greater than 60% fertilization rate was achieved with semen parameters that would have been considered hopeless for IVF (Table 1). Accordingly, ICSI has been described as 'the greatest advance since IVF'.

The main concern about this technique has been whether damage caused by direct injection might lead to an increased chance of chromosomal, particularly sex-chromosomal, abnormalities and malformations in the babies (7). Results from recent large series of procedures have been reassuring (8, 9), but attention now focuses on the male karyotype. Chromosomal anomalies microdeletions have been identified in about 10% of severely oligospermic men (10).

Table 1 European success rates with ICSI up to 1994

Variable	Number	%
Treatment cycles	10 335	-
Oocytes injected	86 165	-
Oocytes fertilized	52 392	60.8% of oocytes injected
Total embryo transfers	9 581	92.7% of cycles
Frozen embryo transfers	2 374	23.0% of cycles
Viable pregnancies	2 139	20.7% of cycles

Testicular failure

Sperm donation is an established and successful technique; typical pregnancy rates are 70% at 12 cycles. Freezing and banking sperm from male patients about to undergo cytotoxic cancer therapy is common practice. Sperm from adolescent boys (14-17 years) is comparable with that of older men in terms of concentration and motility, but for younger children cryopreservation of testicular biopsies has great potential; pregnancies have already been achieved with frozen--thawed sperm extracted from adult testicular tissue. A storm of controversy has arisen over the use of testicular biopsy and immature sperm for ICSI, and a moratorium on its use is in force in the UK, because of anxieties about risks of chromosomal abnormalities in the offspring.

Ovarian failure, egg donation and hormonal replacement

The diagnoses resulting in gonadal failure that require egg donation therapy are shown in Table 2. This technique has been marvellously successful during the last 10 years.

Table 2 Causes of ovarian failure

Chromosal anomalies (particularly Turner's syndrome)
XX gonadal dysgenesis
Childhood radiotherapy/chemotherapy
Autoimmune disorders
Galactosaemia

The principle of treatment is to create an artificial menstrual cycle by using hormone supplements, followed by the timed transfer of donated eggs or embryos. The original hormone replacement regimen by Lutjen in Australia in 1984 (11) was an attempt to mimic a natural menstrual cycle by escalating doses of oestradiol, followed by the addition of progestogen in the luteal phase. In practice, most units now use a supraphysiological regimen, with the aim of transforming the endometrium from an atrophic to a secretory phase.

The success rate in women with Turner's syndrome appears to be particularly good; British data suggest a 25% success rate. Overall, the national British data for oocyte donation indicate a 20% pregnancy rate. Conversely, women who have undergone abdominal irradiation in childhood have poor results from oocyte donation. Critchley *et al.* (12) found that such women had poor uterine arterial blood flow, and a smaller uterus and less responsive endometrium than normal. In addition, retrospective data from a survey of survivors of childhood cancer showed that, for those who had received radiotherapy, mostly for Wilms' tumour, the first pregnancy had an elevated risk of spontaneous abortion and a highly significantly reduced birthweight (both presumably due to radiation-induced structural changes).

Oocyte donation

Donors

This technique is not widely available, partly because of the cost, but partly also because of the shortage of oocyte donors; the oocyte donor must undergo a stimulated gonadotrophin cycle, and a surgical procedure to collect the eggs. In Britain alone about 2000 couples are waiting for oocyte donation, and the waiting time is 1-2 years.

In Britain most donors are anonymous volunteers; this is generally considered preferable to 'known donors', relatives or close friends of the receiving couple. It is not difficult to imagine some of the ethical dilemmas involved when the genetic mother of the child is the familial aunt. IVF patients have been used as a convenient source of donations, but that may affect the patient's own chance of success: in giving away her spare eggs, the patient will have fewer for freezing. Sterilization patients constitute a possible source of oocytes. Offering a free cycle to IVF oocyte donors and paying anonymous donors are not acceptable in Britain, although the latter is the norm in the USA. The ethics of inducement to donate eggs is a matter of debate.

Other sources of oocytes

The shortage of oocyte donors has led to investigation of other potential sources of donations from ovarian grafts, cadaver material and fetal ovaries. Fetal material harvested from mid-trimester terminations is less immunogenic than grafts from adults. The UK Human Fertilization and Embryology Authority's 1994 consultation document (13) led to widespread public debate, and the method was banned in the UK. Oocyte cryopreservation and maturation of immature eggs *in vitro* are two further techniques that could help the overcome the current shortage; it has proved extremely difficult to freeze the mature oocyte successfully, and hopes are being pinned on the latter technique. Eggs can be harvested from donors in natural unstimulated cycles, so avoiding the risks of gonadotrophin treatment. Trounson *et al.* (14) retrieved around 15 oocytes/cycle from women with polycystic ovaries; four-fifths reached metaphase II, one-third of these were fertilized, of which half developed into embryos. One of 13 embryo transfers resulted in pregnancy.

The technique of ovarian tissue cryopreservation has a long history in animal work, with successful pregnancies from frozen-thawed ovarian grafts in mammals. Ovarian biopsy for storage is now being offered to women about to undergo cancer therapy. In future, the thawed ovarian tissue might be reimplanted into a site suitable for revascularization and accessible for egg collection. Alternatively, immature oocytes may be harvested from the thawed tissue and developed for fertilization *in vitro*.

Postscript

The speed of progress in the last 5 years of developments in reproductive technology has astounded even those working in the field. This chapter has indicated some future possibilities. Many raise difficult moral and ethical questions. Doctors and researchers working in the field of human fertility in Britain have legal responsibilities to the regulatory body, the Human Fertilization and Embryology Authority. Such workers everywhere have responsibilities to provide information to the public and to patients.

References

1   Hull MGR, Glazener CMA, Kelly NJ, Conway DI, Foster PA, Hinton RA, Coulson C, Lambert PA, Watt EM, & Desai KM. Population study of causes, treatment, and outcome of infertility. *British Medical Journal* 1985 **291** 1693-1697.

2   Botting BJ. Reproductive trends in the UK. In: *Infertility*, pp 3-21. Eds AA Templeton & JO Drife. London: Springer-Verlag, 1992.

3   Rossing MA, Daling JR, Weiss NS, Moore DE, & Self SG. Ovarian tumours in a cohort of infertile women. *New England Journal of Medicine* 1994 **331** 771-776.

4   Donesky BW & Adashi EY. Surgically induced ovulation in the polycystic ovary syndrome: wedge resection revisited in the age of laparoscopy. *Fertility and Sterility* 1995 **63** 439-463.

5   Federman DD. Psychosexual adjustment in congenital adrenal hyperplasia. *New England Journal of Medicine* 1987 **316** 209-211.

6   Mulaikal RM, Migeon CJ & Rock JA. Fertility rates in female patients with congenital adrenal hyperplasia due to 21-hydroxylase deficiency. *New England Journal of Medicine* 1987 **316** 178-182.

7   In't Veld P, Brandenburg H, Verhoeff A, Dhont M & Los F. Sex chromosomal abnormalities and intra-cytoplasmic sperm injection. *Lancet* 1995 **346** 773.

8   Bonduelle M, Legein J, Buysse A, Van Assche E, Wisanto A, Devroey P, Van Steirteghem AC & Liebaers I. Prospective follow-up study of 423 children born after intra-cytoplasmic sperm injection. *Human Reproduction* 1996 11 1558-1564.

9   Wennerholm UP, Bergh C, Hamberger L, Nilsson L, Reismer E, Wennergren M & Wikland M. Obstetric and perinatal outcome of pregnancies following intracytoplasmic sperm injection. *Human Reproduction* 1996 **11** 1113-1119.

10   Kent-First MG, Kol S, Muallem A, Ofir R, Manor D, Blazer S, First N & Itskovitz-Eldor J. The incidence and possible relevance of Y-linked microdeletions in babies born after intracytoplasmic sperm injection and their infertile fathers. *Molecular human Reproduction* 1996 **2** 943-950.

11   Lutjen P, Trounson A, Leeton J, Findlay J, Wood C & Renou P. The establishment and maintenance of pregnancy using *in vitro* fertilization and embryo donation in a patient with primary ovarian failure. *Nature* 1984 **307** 174-175.

12   Critchley HOD, Wallace WHB, Shalet SM, Mamtora H, Higginson J & Anderson DC. Abdominal irrradiation in childhood: the potential for pregnancy. *British Journal of Obstetrics and Gynaecology* 1992 **99** 392-394.

13   Human Fertilisation and Embryology Authority. *Donated Ovarian Tissue in Embryo Research and Assisted Conception.* London: HFEA 1994.

14   Trounson A, Wood C & Kausche A. *In vitro* maturation and developmental competence of oocytes recovered from untreated polycystic ovarian patients. *Fertility and Sterility* 1994 **62** 353-362.

Virilisation and psychosexual adjustment

Adolescent Endocrinology
Ed R Stanhope
BioScientifica Ltd, Bristol (1998)

Psychosexual development of women with congenital adrenal hyperplasia

K J Zucker

Child and Adolescent Gender Identity Clinic, Child and Family Studies Centre, Clarke Institute of Psychiatry, Toronto, Canada

Models of psychosexual differentiation are presented to aid understanding of the rationale for some of the aspects of psychosexual development that were investigated in a study of women with congenital adrenal hyperplasia (CAH), a family of autosomal recessive disorders of steroid synthesis; CAH is the most common cause of female pseudohermaphroditism (1).

Identity, role and orientation

In the models of psychosexual differentiation, the three major variables are gender identity, gender role, and sexual orientation.

Gender identity

This simple concept relates to a young child's sense of the self as a boy or girl. Many studies of normal development show that children begin to acquire a basic sense of being male or female between 18 months and 3 years of age. Young children are quite aware of phenotypic and social markers that distinguish boys from girls.

Gender role

This term defines behaviours that are culturally characterized as being more typical of masculine or feminine behaviour.

Sexual orientation

This term describes the direction of an individual's erotic attraction, to people of the same sex, the other sex, or both sexes.

Some temporal sequence models of psychosexual differentiation consider gender identity as emerging first, followed by gender role differentiation and then the beginning of the consolidation of sexual orientation at around the time of puberty. However, from the aetiological aspect one can also consider non-temporal models, which are concerned less with the correct sequence than with understanding which factors are related to all three variables.

Most of my clinical and research work at the Gender Identity Clinic in Toronto involves young children who have very severe conflicts in their gender identity development, even though they show no palpable biological anomalies. Examples of psychosexual inversion with regard to gender identity and gender role include a boy who was obsessed with his mother's shoes at 10 months of age, and at 3 years still spends much of his time cross-dressing in women's clothing. His gender identity is clearly female (e.g. he labels himself a girl and indicates that he has a vulva, not a penis). Another example is a 5-year-old girl who wanted a penis for her 5th birthday, and whose phenotypic markers such as hair and clothes are those of a boy. The most extreme instance of cross-gender identification is illustrated by a 19-year-old biological male taking female hormones and undergoing genital surgery.

Normal differentiation and intersex conditions

In the study of psychosexual differentiation in 'normal' children, it has long been recognized that it is very difficult to separate biological and psychosocial factors, because these are typically confounded; and the fact that males are reared as boys and females are reared as girls is often forgotten by psychologists. Normative data (e.g. from Forest (2)) show marked sex differences between males and females with respect to androgen levels in amniotic fluid, particularly for testosterone and Δ-4-androstenedione. These are variables that also may be important in normative psychosexual differentiation.

Physical intersex conditions are important to the understanding of psychosexual differentiation, because with these it is possible to separate biological and psychosocial factors to some extent. Particularly prominent in our field has been the *prenatal hormonal model* of psychosexual differentiation. For decades people have studied the influence of the sex hormones on psychosexual differentiation, and animal models have been particularly helpful for documenting the role of prenatal sex hormones in affecting sex-dimorphic behaviour.

CAH

CAH in women has probably been one of the most interesting intersex conditions to study, because of the very clear evidence of atypical hormone exposure *in utero*.

In about 90% of CAH cases impaired 21-hydroxylase activity in the adrenal cortex leads to cortisol deficiency; in the absence of cortisol feedback, cortisol precursors and androgenic steroids accumulate, and the androgens cause virilization in the genetic female foetus with manifestations ranging from clitoral enlargement to fusion of the labioscrotal folds and a phallic urethra (1, 3).

Forest (2) was able to measure testosterone values in amniotic fluid during at-risk pregnancies and found that the testosterone levels for the affected female foetuses were very close to the normative data on biological males. Not many studies have measured androgen levels in CAH-affected babies directly, but an excessive exposure is inferred from the variable degree of genital masculinization typically seen in affected CAH females.

In early studies the external genitalia were corrected relatively late in development, but in our population surgical cosmesis (clitoral reduction etc.) was performed at a lower median age of 2.5 years (range 2 months-12 years).

Endocrine (cortisone-replacement) therapy for such patients has been available for 40 years; it can control or eliminate postnatal virilization by restricting the anomalous androgen exposure to the prenatal period, but is not always effective in practice (e.g. because of non-compliance).

Salt-wasting and simple virilization in CAH

A distinction has recently been drawn between CAH patients who are simple virilizers (SV) and 'salt wasters' (SW) who have aldosterone deficiency resulting in low serum sodium and high potassium (3). The ratio of SW to SV is about 3:1. Several recent studies have shown that SW are more physically masculinized than SV.

Psychosexual development in female SV and SW CAH patients

We made an adult follow-up psychosexual assessment of female SV and SW patients as part of a larger study of CAH.

Patients

Of 54 genetic female CAH patients identified by searching the records of the Hospital for Sick Children in Toronto, Ontario Canada, 31 participated in the study. Ten individuals (all SW) refused, and 13 were not available. The 22 control subjects (83% participation rate) were the sisters or cousins of the CAH patients. All participants were at least 18 years old (range 18-40 years, patient mean 24 years, control mean 25 years).

Measures

Table 1 shows the six variables in the psychosexual assessment protocol.

Table 1 Variables in the psychosexual assessment protocol for women with CAH

Sex assignment at birth ($\male$, $\female$, delayed assignment)

Recalled childhood gender identity/role

Current gender identity

Marital/relationship status

Current/lifetime sexual orientation in fantasy

Current/lifetime sexual orientation in behaviour (interpersonal sexual experiences with men or women)

Results

CAH subjects vs controls Many free play studies show that girls with CAH prefer to play with stereotypical 'masculine toys', and the CAH subjects in this study also recalled significantly more of such cross-gender behaviour (P=0.009) and identification with the opposite sex (P=0.06) than controls did. They also had fewer exclusively heterosexual fantasies (lifetime rating P=0.02) and sexual experiences with men (lifetime rating P=0.088).

No significant differences were found between CAH and control subjects with respect to dissatisfaction with their sex (gender dysphoria) in adulthood, relationship status (single/in a relationship), or rates of sexual experience with women.

SW vs SV subjects Several significant psychosexual differences emerged between SV and SW. Significantly more of the SW than SV were assigned to the male sex or had delayed assessment of their gender than the SV (P<0.025), possibly suggesting that the SW showed more genital masculinization at birth. (All the male-assigned subjects were reassigned to the female sex at 1-2 months of age.)

SW also recalled more cross-gender behaviour in childhood than SV (P=0.006), were more likely to be single at the time of assessment (P=0.021) and had had fewer sexual experiences with men during the preceding 12 months (P=0.004).

Conclusions

Although the SW-SV differences in this study agreed with some earlier empirical findings (e.g. those of Slijper (4) and Dittmann *et al.* (5)), opinions appear to be divided on the existence of differential prenatal androgenization, and SW and SV may stand on a continuum rather than be discrete categories of disorder. However, our conclusions agree with those of earlier workers, that '...excessive prenatal exposure to androgens shifts psychosexual differentiation to a point somewhere in between a female-typical and a male-typical pattern' (1). Notes of caution, however, are that individual variation was considerable, that differences between CAH subjects and controls, and between SV and SW subjects, did not all achieve significance, and that '... self-report of an atypical sexual orientation might be most susceptible to social desirability factors and thus be an important source of error variance' (1).

References

1   Zucker KJ, Bradley SJ, Oliver G, Blake J, Fleming S & Hood J. Psychosexual development of women with congenital adrenal hyperplasia. *Hormones and Behaviour* 1996 **30** 300-318.

2   Forest MG. Pitfalls in prenatal diagnosis of 21-hydroxylase deficiency by amniotic fluid steroid analysis? A six years experience in 102 pregnancies at risk. *Annals of the New York Academy of Science* 1985 **458** 130-147.

3   New MI, Ghizzoni L & Speiser PW. Update on congenital adrenal hyperplasia. In: *Pediatric Endocrinology,* edn 3, pp 305-320. Ed F Lifshitz. New York: Marcel Dekker, 1996.

4   Slijper FME. Androgens and gender role behaviour in girls with congenital adrenal hyperplasia. (CAH). *Progress in Brain Research* 1984 **61** 417-422.

5   Dittmann RW, Kappes MH, Kappes ME, Börger D, Meyer-Bahlburg HFL *et al.* Congenital adrenal hyperplasia II: gender-related behavior and attitudes in female salt-wasting and simple-virilizing patients. *Psychoneuroendocrinology* 1990 **15** 421-434.

The adrenal, the ovary and hirsutism

Adolescent Endocrinology
Ed R Stanhope
BioScientifica Ltd, Bristol (1998)

The clinical spectrum of congenital adrenal hyperplasia in adolescence and adulthood

R Azziz

Department of Obstetrics and Gynaecology and Medicine,
University of Alabama at Birmingham, Birmingham, AL, USA

Classical and 'non-classical' congenital adrenal hyperplasia (CAH and NCAH) are both part of a continuum of 21-hydroxylase deficiency, including the salt-wasting (salt-losing) form and the simple virilizing form with or without plasma renin increase (Fig. 1). CAH is one of the most common autosomal recessive disorders known, and most studies in the USA show a prevalence of 1-2% for NCAH among hyperandrogenic women; in continental Europe the figures are around 4-6%, and in the Middle and Far East, 6-8%. Prevalence of NCAH among children with premature pubarche is generally low in the USA (0-6%), but higher (up to 20%) in some Latin countries. Patients with NCAH usually present with short stature and mild features of androgen excess which first appear peripubertally, often coinciding with adrenarche; they include acne, androgenic alopecia, hirsutism and oligo-ovulation.

NCAH

The severity of NCAH varies generally according to the age at presentation (Fig. 1).

Genetic basis

The 21-hydroxylase gene, *CYP21*, is located on the short arm of chromosome 6. One of the reasons why CAH is so common is that a pseudogene downstream from it causes a number of mutations by gene conversion. About 14 mutations of the 21-hydroxylase gene, with mild or serious effects, have been described (1).

Two genetic concepts are particularly important in understanding CAH in general. One is that individuals carry more than one gene defect, so that they can be both affected by, and carriers of, different forms of CAH. The individual with NCAH may have a mild mutation inherited from each parent, or have one mild and one severe mutation; and even in so-called 'homozygous' individuals, the two gene defects may not be identical. Hence, because of the great variety of mutations, most individuals carrying gene defects are 'compound heterozygotes'. The variety of gene defects and combinations of defects also means that devising a single genetic screening panel is difficult.

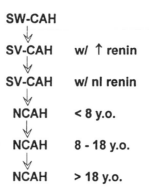

Fig. 1 The continuum of 21-hydroxylase deficiency disorders, from salt-wasting (SW) CAH through the simple virilizing (SV) form to NCAH. y.o., years old.

Diagnosis

Clinical presentation Of 117 women in a recent multicentre study (mean age 25 years), hirsutism was a presenting feature in 82%, oligomenorrhoea in about 50%, acne in 25% and infertility in 10%; alopecia and primary amenorrhoea were also present in a small proportion of the women (2).

However, the clinical presentation cannot be used to distinguish NCAH from polycystic ovary syndrome (PCOS). Data from Kuttenn *et al.* (3) on 24 women with NCAH illustrate that levels of testosterone and androstenedione are of little diagnostic value in NCAH patients. Although dehydro-epiandrosterone sulphate (DHEAS) is considered one of the unique markers of adrenocortical androgen secretion, DHEAS levels are generally not elevated in patients with NCAH, or no more elevated than in patients with PCOS (3). In effect, DHEAS levels cannot be used to screen for NCAH, and attempting to do so is a common cause of false-negative misdiagnosis.

Endocrine diagnosis The only endocrine parameters of clinical diagnostic utility are basal and stimulated serum 17-hydroxyprogesterone (17-HP) levels. Acute adrenocorticotrophin (ACTH) stimulation tests in NCAH individuals result in a 17-HP level that is significantly different from that of control subjects. The widely used nomogram of New *et al.* (4) essentially indicates that the higher the basal level of 17-HP the higher the stimulated level will be. Their data suggests that about 20ng/ml is the lower limit for NCAH after stimulation. However, on the basis of our own data (5), and those of Kuttenn *et al.*(3) and Dewailly *et al.*(6), the diagnostic criterion for homozygous NCAH individuals can be as low as a level of 17-HP of 10ng/ml.

The specific genotype within NCAH patients correlates loosely with their stimulated 17-HP level: and our work on sibling pairs, assumed to have the same genetic defect, confirms this. Some clinical consequences of this are that, in a more severely affected paediatric population, or among families of classically affected individuals, 17-HP levels will be higher; conversely in a gynaecological population of women with a milder disorder and later presentation, 17-HP levels will be lower.

We take 10ng/ml as our diagnostic limit for NCAH, although this is itself an unusual value; of 111 NCAH subjects recently assessed, only 8% had 17-HP values of 10-14ng/ml, while nearly 80% had values over 20ng/ml (2).

The endocrine criteria for NCAH should not be applied rigidly. Table 1 summarizes the approximate risk of an individual having NCAH according to their stimulated 17-HP level. Those with stimulated 17-HP levels of 10-15ng/ml have a 20-50% chance of being carriers for CAH, the proportions differing according to the population studied. Individuals with values of less than 10ng/ml do not in general have NCAH. A recent study on eight such individuals found that six were carriers for 21-hydroxylase deficiency, but none was homozygously affected (7). Patients with stimulated 17-HP values of 15-200ng/ml are highly likely to have NCAH, and those with values above 200ng/ml generally do not have NCAH, but are affected with simple virilizing or salt-wasting CAH.

It should be noted that the often used diagnostic criterion for NCAH first published by Migeon and colleagues (8), the change in 17-HP level plus the change in progesterone (P4) level divided by the time over which the change is measured ((Δ17-HP+ΔP4)/time of test), is not valid. In fact, this test was designed to detect carriers for CAH, and not patients with NCAH.

Table 1 Approximate probability of diagnosing NCAH according to stimulated 17-HP level

Stimulated 17-HP level	Probability of NCAH (%)
<10 ng/ml (30 nmol/l)	<5
10-15 ng/ml (30-45 nmol/l)	20-50
>15 ng/ml (>45 nmol/l)	>95
>20 ng/ml (>605 nmol/l)	<10

Other diagnostic indicators It is not necessary to perform an ACTH stimulation test on all patients suspected of having NCAH. A basal 17-HP level of less than 2ng/ml generally excludes NCAH with 97-100% negative predictive value (5). However, the positive predictive value of a basal 17-HP level over 2ng/ml is only about 11.5% (R Azziz & LA Hincapie, unpublished results). Patients with a basal 17-HP of less than 2 ng/ml in the follicular phase and in the morning should undergo an acute ACTH test.

It is important to measure basal 17-HP levels in the morning, and in the follicular phase or after a withdrawal bleed. Levels are greater during the luteal phase, giving a false-positive result, and may be below 2ng/ml in the afternoon.

Cost of diagnosis Using the basal 17-HP level as a screening tool, R Azziz and LA Hincapie (unpublished data) have estimated the cost per case diagnosed to be about $3500-$7500 in Birmingham, Alabama, USA, where the incidence of NCAH among hyperandrogenic women is approximately 2%. The cost would be lower in areas of the world where the prevalence of NCAH is higher (e.g. Europe, the Middle East).

Development of hyperandrogenism

How do patients become hyperandrogenic? The mechanisms of steroid excess include adrenocortical excess, ovarian excess and possibly peripheral metabolism of 17-HP and P4 to androgens. As the work of Levin *et al.* (9) has shown, older patients with NCAH tend to develop a PCOS-like picture after many years of adrenocortical androgen excess. In these patients with NCAH it becomes difficult to distinguish whether the androgen excess is purely adrenal or adrenal and ovarian.

The excess of adrenal androgens may arise by several possible mechanisms (Table 2). The classic picture is that deficient cortisol production does not properly inhibit pituitary ACTH secretion. ACTH levels then increase, causing hyperplasia of the adrenal leading to increased adrenal androgen production to compensate for the decreased cortisol. This mechanism operates in virtually all cases of classic CAH and about 40% of NCAH. However, Feuillan *et al.* (10) found no measurable excess of serum ACTH, or lower cortisol in relation to ACTH, in most patients with NCAH compared with normal subjects.

Table 2 Mechanisms of adrenocortical androgen excess in CAH and NCAH

Mechanism	Frequency in:	
	CAH	NCAH
Increased ACTH stimulation in response to inadequate cortisol	All	40%
Altered 21-hydroxylase kinetics increasing precursor/product ratios independent of degree of ACTH stimulation	All	All
Physiological inefficiency of $P450_{17\alpha}$ for 17-HP and other Δ^4 steroids	All	All
Compensatory overactivity of other steroidogenic steps	?	?

Changes in the kinetics of 21-hydroxylase, the physiological inefficiency of cytochrome $P450a_{17\alpha}$ for Δ^4 steroids, and compensatory overactivity of other steroidogenic steps are other possible mechanisms (Table 2).

Fertility in simple and salt-wasting CAH

Fertility rate is much lower in women with salt-wasting CAH than simple CAH (e.g. zero vs 60% term pregnancies respectively (11)). Although ovulation can be induced in salt-wasters, other problems preventing conception and term delivery include an inadequate vaginal introitus (even after surgical repair), excessive secretion of progesterone resulting in ovulatory dysfunction, inadequacies of the endometrium, poor cervical mucus, and possibly poor oocyte quality.

Treatment of symptoms of CAH

A symptom of major psychosocial importance to affected women is hirsutism, and antiandrogens are the treatment of choice. In fact, glucocorticoid treatment alone in women with NCAH has less of an impact on hair growth than does the addition of an antiandrogen (12).

References

1   Azziz R, Dewailly D & Owerbach D. Non-classic adrenal hyperplasia: Current concepts. *Journal of Clinical Endocrinology and Metabolism* 1994 **78** 810-815.

2   Knochenhauer ES, Waggoner WT, Azziz R, Carmina E, Dewailly D, Fruzzetti F, Ibanez L, Marcondes JAM, Mendonca BB, Rohmer V, Speiser PW & Zacur HA. Clinical features and genotype of 21-hydroxylase (21-OH) deficient non-classic adrenal hyperplasia (NCAH): A multicenter study. The 79th Annual Meeting of the Endocrine Society, Minneapolis, MN, June 11-14 1997 1-358.

3   Kuttenn F, Couillin P, Girard F, Billaud L, Vincens M, Bouchkkine C, *et al.* Late-onset adrenal hyperplasia in hirsutism. *New England Journal of Medicine* 1985 **313** 224-231.

4   New MI, Lorenzen F, Lerner AJ, *et al.* Genotyping steroid 21-hydroxylase deficiency: hormonal reference data. *Journal of Clinical Endocrinology and Metabolism* 1983 **57** 320-326.

5   Azziz R & Zacur HA. 21-Hydroxylase deficiency in female hyperandrogenemia: Screening and diagnosis. *Journal of Clinical Endocrinology and Metabolism* 1989 **69** 577-578.

6   Dewailly D, Vantyghem-Haudiquet MC, Sainsard C *et al.* Clinical and biological phenotypes in late-onset 21-hydroxylase deficiency. *Journal of Clinical Endocrinology and Metabolism* 1986 **63** 418-423.

7   Azziz R & Owerbach D. Molecular abnormalities of the 21-hydroxylase gene in hyperandrogenic women with an exaggeratee 17-hydroxprogesterone response to acute adrenal stimulation. *American Journal of Obstetrics and Gynecology* 1995 **172** 914-918.

8   Gutai JP, Kowarski AA & Migeon CJ. The detection of the heterozygote carrier for congenital virilizing adrenal hyperplasia. *Journal of Pediatrics* 1977 **90** 924-929.

9   Levin JH, Carmina E & Lobo RA. Is the inappropriate gonoadotropin secretion of patients with polycystic ovary syndrome similar to that of patients with adult-onset congential adrenal hyperplasia? *Fertility and Sterility* 1991 **56** 635-640.

10   Feuillan P, Pang S, Schürmeyer T, Avgerinos PC & Chrousos GP. The hypothalamic-pituitary-adrenal axis in partial (late-onset) 21-hydroxylase deficiency. *Journal of Clinical Endocrinology and Metabolism* 1988 **67** 154-160.

11   Mulaikal RM, Migeon CJ & Rock JA. Fertility rates in females patients with congenital adrenal hyperplasia due to 21-hydroxylase deficiency. *New England Journal of Medicine* 1987 **326** 178-182.

12   Spritzer P, Billaud L, Thalabard JC *et al.* Cyproterone acetate versus hydrocortisone treatment in late-onset adrenal hyperplasia. *Journal of Clinical Endocrinology and Metabolism* 1990 **70** 642-646.

Adolescent Endocrinology
Ed R Stanhope
BioScientifica Ltd, Bristol (1998)

Long-term sequelae of premature adrenarche and pubarche

L Ibáñez and N Potau

Adolescent and Endocrinology Unit, Hospital Materno-Infantil Vall
d'Hebron, Universitat Autònoma, Barcelona, Spain

Adrenarche is the increase in adrenal androgen secretion that begins at about 6 years of chronological age. During adrenarche the adrenal cortex develops the ability to secrete androgens, probably mainly through increased 17, 20-lyase activity of cytochrome $P450c_{17\alpha}$. This could be due to the activity of a serine-phosphorylation factor, and insulin-like growth factor-I (IGF-I) has been proposed as the trigger for phosphorylation, because its fluctuations in level parallel those of dehydroepiandrosterone (DHEA) and DHEA sulphate (DHEAS). Figure 1 summarizes the core steroidogenic pathway which is common to both the adrenal glands and the ovaries. Cholesterol is converted to pregnenolone by side-chain cleavage, and then to DHEA, principally by a two-step conversion involving cytochrome $P450c_{17\alpha}$.

Premature pubarche (PP)

PP is defined as the early appearance of pubic hair before the age of 8 in girls and the age of 9 in boys, with or without axillary hair and apocrine pubertal odour, and with no other signs of sexual development. PP occurs much more frequently in males than in females, and is usually secondary to premature adrenarche. Adrenal androgens, particularly DHEA, androstenedione and testosterone, are moderately increased for chronological age, but fall within the range expected from the Tanner pubic hair stage. However, in up to one quarter of patients with isolated or typical PP, DHEAS levels are even higher than those corresponding to normal children matched for bone age or pubic hair stage (Fig. 2) (1).

Congenital adrenal hyperplasia (CAH)

PP can be the first sign of late-onset CAH. The frequency of CAH among patients with PP differs in different populations; in Spain it is about 7%. Our diagnostic policy is to perform an adrenocorticotrophin test for CAH only in girls who have elevated levels of androgens other than DHEAS. If only DHEAS is elevated and there are no signs suggesting atypical PP (e.g. clitoral enlargement, advanced bone age), the presumptive diagnosis is idiopathic PP.

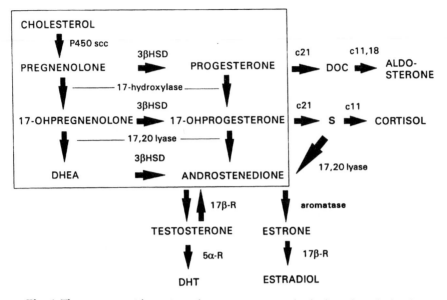

Fig. 1 The core steroidogenic pathway common to both the adrenal glands and the ovaries. DHT, dihydrotestosterone; scc, side-chain cleavage; 3βHSD, 3β-hydroxysteroid dehydrogenase; 17β-R, 17β-reductase; 5α-R, 5α-reductase, DOC, deoxycorticosterone, S, 11-deoxycortisol. Reproduced with permission from (8).

Isolated PP

Our first study investigating outcomes in isolated PP was undertaken in conjunction with the Italian group of Dr R Virdis in Parma, Italy (2). The populations from the two centres had comparable characteristics. Of 127 girls diagnosed with isolated PP, 69 had begun puberty, 49 had had menarche, and 38 had attained final height. Ovarian function was assessed in 35. Advanced skeletal maturation and tall stature were constant features during the early years of follow-up, but declined progressively later. Gonadarche began at a mean age of 9.7 years, and menarche occurred at 12.0 years, which is no different from maternal and population mean menarcheal ages (Table 1).

Girls in both populations followed the normal secular trend for height. Their final heights (mean 160 cm) were correlated with height prognosis at diagnosis and onset of puberty, and were greater than parental heights. We concluded from this auxological study that PP produced a transient acceleration in growth and bone maturation, with no deleterious effects on the onset of puberty or on final height.

Although these results appeared reassuring, we were still concerned about the potential later effects of PP on ovarian function, the possibility having been raised that individuals with PP may have an increased incidence of hirsutism and polycystic ovary syndrome (PCOS).

Adolescent Endocrinology
Ed R Stanhope
BioScientifica Ltd, Bristol (1998)

Long-term sequelae of premature adrenarche and pubarche

L Ibáñez and N Potau

Adolescent and Endocrinology Unit, Hospital Materno-Infantil Vall d'Hebron, Universitat Autònoma, Barcelona, Spain

Adrenarche is the increase in adrenal androgen secretion that begins at about 6 years of chronological age. During adrenarche the adrenal cortex develops the ability to secrete androgens, probably mainly through increased 17, 20-lyase activity of cytochrome $P450c_{17\alpha}$. This could be due to the activity of a serine-phosphorylation factor, and insulin-like growth factor-I (IGF-I) has been proposed as the trigger for phosphorylation, because its fluctuations in level parallel those of dehydroepiandrosterone (DHEA) and DHEA sulphate (DHEAS). Figure 1 summarizes the core steroidogenic pathway which is common to both the adrenal glands and the ovaries. Cholesterol is converted to pregnenolone by side-chain cleavage, and then to DHEA, principally by a two-step conversion involving cytochrome $P450c_{17\alpha}$.

Premature pubarche (PP)

PP is defined as the early appearance of pubic hair before the age of 8 in girls and the age of 9 in boys, with or without axillary hair and apocrine pubertal odour, and with no other signs of sexual development. PP occurs much more frequently in males than in females, and is usually secondary to premature adrenarche. Adrenal androgens, particularly DHEA, androstenedione and testosterone, are moderately increased for chronological age, but fall within the range expected from the Tanner pubic hair stage. However, in up to one quarter of patients with isolated or typical PP, DHEAS levels are even higher than those corresponding to normal children matched for bone age or pubic hair stage (Fig. 2) (1).

Congenital adrenal hyperplasia (CAH)

PP can be the first sign of late-onset CAH. The frequency of CAH among patients with PP differs in different populations; in Spain it is about 7%. Our diagnostic policy is to perform an adrenocorticotrophin test for CAH only in girls who have elevated levels of androgens other than DHEAS. If only DHEAS is elevated and there are no signs suggesting atypical PP (e.g. clitoral enlargement, advanced bone age), the presumptive diagnosis is idiopathic PP.

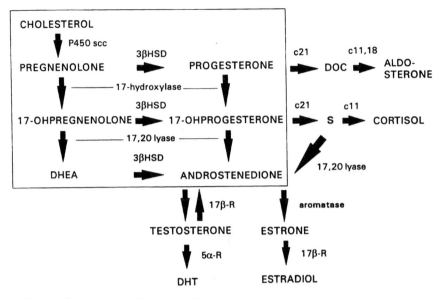

Fig. 1 The core steroidogenic pathway common to both the adrenal glands and the ovaries. DHT, dihydrotestosterone; scc, side-chain cleavage; 3βHSD, 3β-hydroxysteroid dehydrogenase; 17β-R, 17β-reductase; 5α-R, 5α-reductase, DOC, deoxycorticosterone, S, 11-deoxycortisol. Reproduced with permission from (8).

Isolated PP

Our first study investigating outcomes in isolated PP was undertaken in conjunction with the Italian group of Dr R Virdis in Parma, Italy (2). The populations from the two centres had comparable characteristics. Of 127 girls diagnosed with isolated PP, 69 had begun puberty, 49 had had menarche, and 38 had attained final height. Ovarian function was assessed in 35. Advanced skeletal maturation and tall stature were constant features during the early years of follow-up, but declined progressively later. Gonadarche began at a mean age of 9.7 years, and menarche occurred at 12.0 years, which is no different from maternal and population mean menarcheal ages (Table 1).

Girls in both populations followed the normal secular trend for height. Their final heights (mean 160 cm) were correlated with height prognosis at diagnosis and onset of puberty, and were greater than parental heights. We concluded from this auxological study that PP produced a transient acceleration in growth and bone maturation, with no deleterious effects on the onset of puberty or on final height.

Although these results appeared reassuring, we were still concerned about the potential later effects of PP on ovarian function, the possibility having been raised that individuals with PP may have an increased incidence of hirsutism and polycystic ovary syndrome (PCOS).

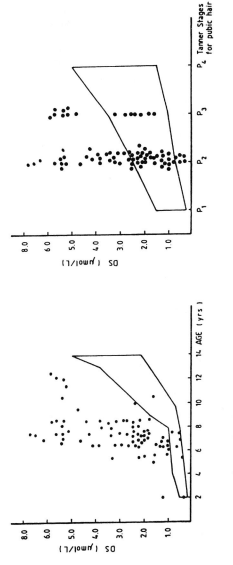

Fig. 2 Plasma levels of DHEAS (DS) in girls with PP compared with age-matched (left) and Tanner pubertal stage-matched control values (right), indicated by outlines. Redrawn with permission from (1).

Table 1 Chronological and bone age at onset of puberty (Tanner breast stage 2 (B2)), menarche and maternal and population menarcheal ages in two Latin populations (Northern Italian and Northern Spanish) of girls with PP. Values are the mean±S.D.

	CA at B2 (years)	BA at B2 (years)	Menarche (years)	Maternal menarche (years)	Population menarche (years)
Parma	9.4±1.0 (n=32)	10.7±0.6 (n=32)	12.0±1.2 (n=17)	12.2±1.7 (n=17)	12.4±1.0 (n=1260)
Barcelona	9.9±1.0 (n=37)	11.3±0.9 (n=37)	12.0±0.9 (n=25)	12.6±1.8 (n=25)	12.3±0.7 (n=1861)
Total	9.7±0.9 (n=69)	11.0±1.0 (n=69)	12.0±1.0 (n=42)	12.5±1.8 (n=42)	12.3±0.8 (n=3121)

CA, chronological age; BA, bone age; B2, Tanner breast stage 2. Data from (2).

Late effects of PP

To investigate this, 27 girls (age 14±1.5 years) with a history of PP due to premature adrenarche received an ultrasound scan and were screened for hirsutism, menstrual disturbance and baseline androgen levels. To our surprise, 9/27 were hirsute, many had elevated baseline androgen levels, three were oligomenorrhoeic, and three had PCOS on ultrasound together with elevated luteinizing hormone/follicle-stimulating hormone (LH/FSH) ratios. Ovarian function in these patients was assessed by the method of Rosenfield *et al.* (3) using a gonadotrophin-releasing hormone (GnRH) agonist to categorize the pituitary-gonadal secretion; such agents produce sequential stimulation of the pituitary (maximum stimulation up to 4 h after the challenge) and the gonads (16-24 h).

Rosenfield *et al.* used the GnRH analogue nafarelin in a group of women with classical PCOS, a group of normal women and a group of normal men. They found that 17-hydroxyprogesterone secretion in response to the agonist was significantly higher in women with PCOS than in normal women, being actually within the male range. They hypothesized that this exaggerated response could be due to dysregulation of cytochrome $P450c_{17\alpha}$ in the ovary, particularly its 17, 20-lyase activity.

Functional ovarian hyperandrogenism (FOH)

Such studies led to the concept of functional ovarian hyperandrogenism; individuals with this diagnosis include those who show a PCOS-type response to a GnRH analogue, who have hyperandrogenaemia, hirsutism or menstrual disturbances, but who do not necessarily meet all the criteria for classical PCOS (e.g. polycystic ovaries on ultrasound and an elevated LH/FSH ratio). According to Rosenfield *et al.* (3). FOH is caused by increased intra-ovarian androgen secretion leading to hyperandrogenaemia and follicular atresia. This may be due to extra-ovarian androgen elevation or ovarian steroidogenic blocks, and at the same time to the dysregulation of ovarian androgen secretion. Such dysregulation can arise from elevation of LH levels or augmentation of insulin or other growth factors such as IGF-I (4).

Frequency of FOH

We went on to investigate the frequency of FOH in our population compared with that in the normal population, using the GnRH analogue leuprolide acetate. Thirty-five non-obese 15-year-old girls with PP were compared with 12 age-matched controls. All were 3 years post-menarche. Of the girls with PP, 16 were oligomenorrhoeic, with an elevated hirsutism score, eight had polycystic ovaries on ultrasound, increased LH/FSH ratios and elevated androstenedione or testosterone, and 19 were regularly menstruating and had baseline androgen levels similar to those in the controls. All subjects received a single subcutaneous dose of leuprolide acetate, 500 µg, and the levels of gonadotrophin, androgens and oestrogens before and 24 hours after challenge were assessed (5).

Gonadotrophin levels increased to a similar extent in all three groups (oligomenorrheic, regularly menstruating, controls), but levels of ovarian androgens differed. Androstenedione was clearly more elevated in the oligomenorrhoeics than in the other two groups, but some values overlapped between groups. In the case of 17-hydroxyprogesterone, the response was clearly distinct, with no overlap between groups. Oligomenorrhoeic girls showed ovarian 17-hydroxyprogesterone responses greater than 160 ng/dl, which corresponded to the mean (+2 S.D.) value among controls (5).

It is possible in view of the 17-hydroxyprogesterone hyper-response in the ovary that, as cytochrome $P450c_{17\alpha}$ is encoded by the same gene in the adrenals and gonads, dysregulation of this enzyme may begin in childhood, causing premature adrenarche; the same process in the ovary may then give rise to ovarian hyperandrogenism.

Predictive factors

We sought clues as to which girls would develop ovarian hyperandrogenism in the postpubertal period, and a positive correlation was found between levels of DHEAS and androstenedione at diagnosis of PP and the responses of 17-hydroxyprogesterone to the GnRH agonist. Thus girls with a more exaggerated adrenarcheal response were indeed more likely to develop postpubertal ovarian hyperandrogenism.

The increased incidence of ovarian hyperandrogenism in the cohort of postpubertal patients with PP prompted an investigation into whether this pattern of ovarian androgen hyper-responsiveness may begin before the end of puberty. A GnRH analogue test was performed throughout all stages of pubertal development (Tanner breast stages B2 to B5) in a group of girls with PP. It was found that in the Δ^4 and Δ^5 pathways the responses of DHEA and

17-hydroxyprogesterone were higher, at baseline and at peak response to the agonist, in girls with PP than in normal controls; the incremental increases in response to the agonist were also higher than in controls. This pattern of ovarian androgen hyper-responsiveness appears to begin early in puberty, but is more exaggerated during mid and late puberty.

Triggers for ovarian androgen hyper-responsiveness?

The relationship between hyperinsulinaemia and hyperandrogenism may suggest a possible trigger for ovarian androgen hyper-responsiveness. Hyperinsulinaemia and/or insulin resistance and adrenal hyperandrogenism are common features in women and adolescents with classical PCOS and also in FOH. It has been proposed that hyperinsulinaemia *per se* causes hyperandrogenism, and it has been shown that insulin infusions may augment adrenal steroidogenesis in hyperandrogenic women, probably by increasing cytochrome $P450c_{17\alpha}$ activity. It is also well known that insulin modulates IGF-I and IGFBP-1 action, and inhibits sex-hormone-binding globulin production in human hepatoma cell lines, and that there is an inverse relationship between insulin and sex-hormone-binding globulin in normal women. So hyperinsulinaemia is a leading candidate for the cause of dysregulation of androgen secretion in ovarian and adrenal hyperandrogenism.

The defects producing insulin resistance in PCOS appear to be genetic and to be associated with increased serine phosphorylation of the insulin receptor, and a single factor causing serine phosphorylation of the insulin receptor and of ovarian cytochrome $P450c_{17\alpha}$ could produce both insulin resistance and the hyperandrogenism characteristic of PCOS.

Thus the hypothesis is that, while normal adrenal phosphorylation may be triggered during normal adrenarche, abnormal activation of this process can produce both ovarian and adrenal hyperandrogenism and abnormal serine phosphorylation of insulin receptors, leading to hyperinsulinaemia and insulin resistance usually associated with many types of adrenal and ovarian hyperandrogenism.

Insulin secretion patterns in PP

A study of the patterns of insulin secretion in girls with PP seems to support this hypothesis (6). We studied 24 postpubertal girls with PP, 13 of whom had ovarian hyperandrogenism and 11 had not, plus 21 controls. As Figure 3 shows, mean serum insulin (MSI) levels were significantly elevated in patients with PP and FOH compared with controls ($P<0.01$) and were intermediate in patients with PP and not FOH. Insulin sensitivity index (SI) calculated by the method of Cederholm & Wibell (7) did not differ significantly between the three groups.

The hyperinsulinaemia was directly related to the free androgen index, so the greater the hyperandrogenism, the greater the hyperinsulinaemia (6). Oral glucose tolerance tests in prepubertal and pubertal patients with PP and controls showed that MSI was significantly increased relative to controls, and

IGF-I values depressed before puberty and at all pubertal stages. These findings suggest that hyperinsulinaemia and premature adrenarche are pathogenetically linked, and support the concept of a common trigger for the two events.

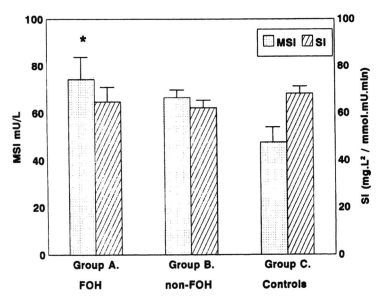

Fig. 3 MSI levels and peripheral insulin SI (means±S.E.M.) in postpubertal girls with PP and FOH (Group A), postpubertal girls with PP but without FOH (Group B) and control subjects (Group C). Redrawn with permission from (5).

Cardiovascular risk

Hyperinsulinaemia has been deemed an independent risk factor for developing cardiovascular disease, and this purported pathogenetic role of insulin can be enhanced by other coexisting factors, such as dyslipidaemia. Preliminary studies show that an increase in triglyceride levels between stages B2 and B5 compared with normal controls is superimposed on the hyperinsulinaemia. Our data suggest that the pattern of atherogenic risk may begin during childhood, and further work is needed in this area.

Conclusions

PP is not necessarily a benign condition, and long-term follow up of these patients is highly recommended, because of the increased incidence of ovarian hyperandrogenism and hyperinsulinaemia. However, neither the genetic basis of this disorder nor the common pathogenesis of hyperandrogenism and hyperinsulinaemia is yet properly understood.

References

1   Virdis R, Zampolli M, Ibáñez I, Ghizzoni L & Vicens-Calvet E. Il pubarca prematuro. *Rivista Italiana di Pediatria* 1993 **19** 569-579.

2   Ibanez L, Virdis R, Potau N, Zampolli M, Ghizzoni L, Albisu MA, Carrascosa A, Bernasconi S & Vicens-Calvet E. Natural history of premature pubarche: An auxological study. *Journal of Clinical Endocrinology and Metabolism* 1992 **74** 254-257.

3   Rosenfield RL, Barnes RB, Cara JF & Lucky AW. Dyregulation of cytochrome P450c17α as the cause of polycystic ovarian syndrome. *Fertility and Sterility* 1990 **53** 785-791.

4   Ehrmann DA, Barnes RB & Rosenfeld RL. Polycystic ovary syndrome as a form of functional ovarian hyperandrogenism due to dysregulation of androgen secretion. *Endocrine Reviews* 1995 **16** 322-353.

5   Ibáñez L, Potau N, Virdis R, Zampolli M, Terzi C, Gussinyé M *et al.* Postpubertal outcome in girls diagnosed with premature pubarche during childhood: increased frequency of functional ovarian hyperandrogenism. *Journal of Clinical Endocrinology and Metabolism* 1993 **76** 1599-1603.

6   Ibanez L, Potau N, Zampolli M, Prat N, Virdis R, Vicens-Calvet E & Carrascosa A. Hyperinsulinaemia in postpubertal girls with a history of premature pubarche and functional ovarian hyperandrogenism. *Journal of Clinical Endocrinology and Metabolism* 1996 **81** 1237-1243.

7   Cederholm J & Wibell L. Insulin release and peripheral insulin sensitivity at the oral glucose tolerance test. *Diabetes Research and Clinical Practice* 1990 **10** 167-175.

8   Rosenfield RL & Lucky AW. Acne, hirsutism and alopecia in adolescent girls. Clinical expression of androgen excess. *Endocrine and Metabolism Clinics of North America* 1993 **22** 507-532

Adolescent Endocrinology
Ed R Stanhope
BioScientifica Ltd, Bristol (1998)

Hirsutism and irregular menses in adolescence

E Porcu and S Venturoli

Institute of Obstetrics and Gynaecology, Reproductive
Endocrinology Unit, University of Bologna, Bologna, Italy

A prospective study which began about 15 years ago aimed to identify the early onset of hyperandrogenic pathology in adolescence, particularly the first steps of the polycystic ovary syndrome (PCOS). Hirsutism and irregular menstrual cycles may be pathological features, but are both very common in normal adolescence. It emerged that menstrual irregularity and subnormal ovulation persisting into adult life leads to a polycystic ovarian transformation with elevated androgen levels.

The study

Our study on girls with irregular menstrual cycles aimed to determine the timing of onset and endocrine and morphological background of hyperandrogenism. More than 100 girls were initially evaluated, and follow-up data over 1-7 years are available on 84 of these. A most surprising finding was that around one-third of the girls had levels of gonadotrophins, particularly luteinizing hormone (LH), testosterone and androstenedione, above the normal adult range (Fig. 1) (1)

Pulsatile gonadotrophin secretion

In anovulatory patients with high LH levels, both frequency and amplitude of secretory pulses were increased, whereas both these parameters were similar to control values in patients with normal LH levels.

Circadian secretory rhythm

Gonadotrophin secretion peaked during the afternoon in anovulatory patients with high LH levels, but during the night in those with normal LH levels (2). Both these patterns in young anovulatory subjects are markedly different from the normal adult pattern, which shows no pronounced circadian fluctuation. High LH levels were associated with high levels of testosterone, dehydrotestosterone and androstenedione.

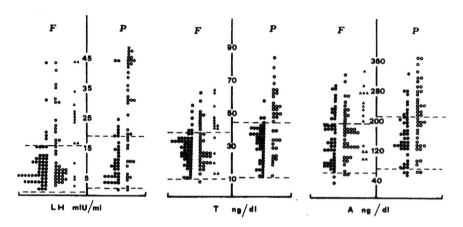

Fig. 1 Distribution of LH, testosterone (T) and androstenedione (A) in amenorrhoeic subjects (▲) on a random day and in subjects with irregular cycles (●, ovulatory; O, anovulatory) during the follicular (F) and the premenstrual (P) phases with reference to the normal adult range (----). The percentages of subjects exceeding the adult range are: for the follicular phase, LH 20%, testosterone 17%, androstenedione 29%; for the premenstrual phase, LH 35.8%, testosterone 26%, androstenedione 33.7%; for amenorrhoeic subjects, LH 73%, testosterone 67%, androstenedione 67%. Reproduced with permission from (1) © S Karger AG, Basel.

Ovarian structure

Transabdominal ultrasonography revealed that adolescent patients with irregular cycles had a greater ovarian volume than those with regular cycles and normal adult controls.

Most patients with irregular cycles also had multiple cystic areas, and the significance of this finding in adolescents is still a matter of debate. The classification of ovarian characteristics developed by Adams and colleagues (3) is presented in Table 1; however, in practice, these characteristics can overlap.

With Adams' classification in mind we performed a detailed analysis of data from our patients. We found that the ovaries were homogeneous in about 36% of patients, multifollicular in 33%, and polycystic in a remarkable 41%. Patients with increased ovarian volume and polycystic ovaries had elevated LH, testosterone and androstenedione levels. We were convinced that LH derangement plays a major role in determining ovarian morphological features.

Origin of polycystic ovaries in adolescents with irregular cycles

Observations on one girl evaluated throughout puberty gave an opportunity to investigate changes in LH secretion and ovarian structure. Early in puberty this subject had a normal pattern of LH secretion and normal ovaries with some

Table 1 Classification of ovarian structure. Reproduced by permission from (3) © The Lancet Ltd.

Ovarian status	Volume	Cystic areas
Homogeneous	Low or normal	<4, ≤5mm
Multifollicular	Normal or high	>5, 5-10 mm, throughout stroma
Polycystic	Normal or high	>10, 3-8 mm, peripheral or central (+ echodense stroma)
Multifollicular or polycystic + dominant follicles	Normal or high	1-2, >13 mm

developing follicles. In mid-puberty the number of developing follicles increased, although the LH pattern was still normal. However, LH levels increased in late puberty, with increased pulse frequency and amplitude, and the ovaries became frankly polycystic.

However, the real cause of PCOS is still obscure. For example, a second girl developed PCOS and hirsutism in late puberty without any abnormality of LH secretion. In addition, Stanhope *et al.* (4) have shown that treatment with pulsatile gonadotrophin-releasing hormone alone in a girl with hypogonadotrophic hypogonadism (and who had therefore not previously been exposed to gonadotrophins) could result in the development of PCOS.

Irregularity and PCOS

Table 2 summarizes the main features of irregular adolescent ovulatory cycles. The similarity of this profile, apart from the absence of hirsutism, to that of PCOS prompted a comparison of such individuals. No significant difference in LH levels was found between the anovulatory girls and patients with PCOS.

Table 2 Main features of adolescent irregular cycles

Characteristics	Incidence (%)
Anovulation	50.9
Enlarged ovaries	46.3
Non-homogeneous ovaries	57.0
High LH levels	30.0
High testosterone and androstenedione levels	30.0

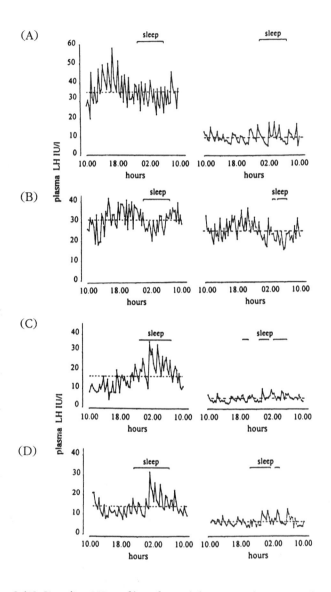

Fig. 2 (A) Circadian LH profiles of an adolescent at the gynaecological age of 3 years (left) and 6 years (right). At the first examination, the subject was anovulatory with high LH levels, whereas she showed an ovulatory cycle at the last evaluation. As a result, the episodic LH secretion showed a decrease in pulse amplitude and frequency and the accentuated circadian variation with the highest levels in the afternoon disappeared. (B) Circadian LH profiles of an adolescent at the gynaecological age of 2 years (left) and 6 years (right). The anovulatory condition with high LH levels of the first examination persisted even later and the episodic and circadian LH patterns did not change except for a slight fall in mean levels. (C) Circadian LH

As to the circadian pattern of LH secretion, patients with PCOS and anovulatory girls with high LH levels had very similar chronobiological patterns (5) by COSINOR analysis (6, 7), which were different from the pattern found in ovulatory subjects. Ovarian volume and structure were slightly different; patients with PCOS had a greater ovarian volume and, by definition, a higher proportion of polycystic ovaries than anovulatory girls with elevated LH.

Progression to PCOS

We posed the question, 'are these girls true candidates to develop PCOS in adult life?', and went on to re-evaluate 84 of our young patients.

The patients

- Mean age 15 (11-19) years
- Follow-up period 1-7 years
- Two to nine examinations
- Mean gynaecological age at first examination 2.7 years
- Mean gynaecological age at last examination 5.5 years

Evidence for progression to PCOS

The first result of this study showed that ovarian volume increased in 30% of patients whose volume was normal at baseline. In addition, some of them developed a polycystic ovarian structure. Conversely, a decrease in ovarian volume was recorded in only 22% of patients who had enlarged ovaries at baseline, and in none of them did the ovarian structure become more normal. In addition, increased ovarian volume and a polycystic structure persisted in over 70% of subjects (8).

Endocrine parameters

Of subjects with normal baseline testosterone values, 31% showed an increase, but a decrease was found in 36% of those who had high initial testosterone levels. In addition, mean LH levels, and pulse amplitude and frequency all fell in about one-third of patients who had had high LH at baseline. In about

profiles of an adolescent at the gynaecological age of 3 years (left) and 5 years (right). At the first examination, the subject was anovulatory with normal LH levels, whereas she showed an ovulatory cycle at the last evaluation. As a result, the accentuated circadian variation with the highest levels in the morning disappeared. (D) Circadian LH profiles of an adolescent at the gynaecological age of 3 years (left) and 6 years (right). The anovulatory condition with normal LH levels of the first examination persisted later. The mean LH levels decreased and the circadian fluctuation was less pronounced even though a nocturnal dominance was still present. Reproduced with permission from (2) © The Endocrine Society.

one-third of patients, the abnormal circadian LH secretory pattern normalized to a smoothed pattern similar to that of normal adult ovulating women (Fig. 2) (9).

Conclusions

A progressive increase in ovulatory frequency leads to normal adult endocrine and morphological structure. However, persistence of anovulation is associated with the establishment of endocrine and morphological features of immaturity which can become pathological as adulthood approaches and are the functional route for the development of hyperandrogenic symptoms. In the adolescent with persistently irregular cycles, long-term anovulation or oligo-ovulation are linked to a progressive increase in ovarian volume and to a polycystic transformation, with increasing androgen levels.

Hyperandrogenaemia is the other side of adolescence. It may sometimes play a physiological role (e.g. in follicular atresia), but this role should be limited. Persistence of hyperandrogenaemia into adulthood may compromise reproductive function. Even in the presence of ablation, hyperandrogenaemia in ovulatory patients may cause reduced fertility, as has been documented by Apter & Vikho (10), and may be the functional basis for androgenic pathology.

Finally, our studies do not lead us to equate hyperandrogenism with hirsutism; the reproductive anomalies of hyperandrogenaemia were only infrequently associated with the clinical manifestation of hirsutism.

References

1   Venturoli S, Porcu E, Fabbri R, Paradisi R, Ruggeri S, Bolelli GF, Orsini LF, Gabbi D, Flamigni C. Menstrual irregularities in adolescents: hormonal pattern and ovarian morphology. *Hormone Research* 1986 **24** 269-279.

2   Porcu E, Venturoli S, MagriniO, Bolzani R, Gabbi D, Paradisi R, Fabbri R, Flamigni C. Circadian variation of luteinizing hormone can have two different profiles in adolescent anovulation. *Journal of Clinical Endocrinology and Metabolism,* 1987 **65** 488-493.

3   Adams J, Polson D, Abdulwahid N, Morrison DV, Franks S, Mason HD, Tucker M, Price J, Jacobs HS. Multifollicular ovaries: clinical and endocrine features and response to pulsatile gonadotropin releasing hormone. *Lancet* 1985 **2** 1375-1378.

4   Stanhope R, Adams J, Pringle JP, Jacobs HS, Brook CGD. The evolution of the polycystic ovaries in a girl with hypogonadotropic hypogonadism before puberty and during puberty induced with pulsatile gonadotropin-releasing hormone. *Fertility and Sterility* 1987 **47** 872-875.

5   Porcu E, Venturoli S & Flamigni C. Relations between puberty and the onset of the polycystic ovary syndrome. In: *Major Advances in Human Female Reproduction* **73**, pp 45-47. Eds EY Adaschi & S Mancuso. New York: Raven Press, 1991.

6   Halberg F, Engeli M, Hamburger C & Hillman D. Spectral resolution of low frequency, small amplitude rhythms in excreted 17-ketosteroids: probable androgen induced circaseptian desynchronization. *Acta Endocrinologica* 1965 **51** (Suppl) 5-13.

7   Bingham L, Arbogast B, Guillaume GC, Lee JK, Halberg F. Inferential statistical methods for estimating and comparing Cosinor parameters. *Chronobiologia* 1982 **9** 397-414.

8   Venturoli S, Porcu E, Fabbri R, Pluchinotta V, Ruggeri S, Macrelli S, Paradisi R, Flamigni C. Longitudinal change of sonographic ovarian aspects and endocrine parameters in irregular cycles of adolescence. *Pediatric Research* 1995 **38** 974-980.

9   Porcu E, Venturoli S, Longhi MP, Fabbri R, Paradisi R, Flamigni C. Chronobiologic evolution of luteinizing hormone secretion in adolescents: developmental patterns and speculation on the onset of the polycystic ovary syndrome. *Fertility and Sterility* 1997 **67** 842-848.

10   Apter D & Vihko R. Endocrine determinants of fertility: serum androgen concenrations during follow up of adolescents into the third decade of life. *Journal of Clinical Endocrinology and Metabolism* 1989 **71** 970-974.

Adolescent Endocrinology
Ed R Stanhope
BioScientifica Ltd, Bristol (1998)

Is polycystic ovary a condition of childhood?

G S Conway

Department of Endocrinology, The Middlesex Hospital, London, UK

The development of polycystic ovary (PCO) in adolescence may be the result of either a genetic programme or environmental factors. Ultrasound has greatly improved our knowledge of PCO in recent years; it becomes apparent on ultrasound at the age of about 6 years, and then becomes more frequent until the adult prevalence of 25% is reached at age 11. Doppler ultrasound demonstrates that blood flow through the ovarian stroma in both PCO and polycystic ovary syndrome (PCOS) is twice as high as that in normal controls. It may be that ovarian angiogenesis precedes any endocrine change in PCO.

Disorders of puberty

Clues about the 'switch' that turns on PCO in a proportion of girls may come from studies of disorders of puberty. Data of Bridges and colleagues (1) suggest that, contrary to expectation, neither premature adrenarche nor premature thelarche predisposes to PCO. However, a very high proportion of young girls who are treated with gonadotrophin-releasing hormone (GnRH) analogues and growth hormone for central precocious puberty develop PCO. Whether this is an effect of growth hormone or a feature of the underlying disorder is not clear.

Congenital adrenal hyperplasia

Most women with congenital adrenal hyperplasia have PCO; among 17 of our patients with the classical form aged between 16 and 46 years, 16 had PCO, and 10 had oligo- or ameno-rrhoea.

Origin of PCOS

Androgen exposure

One view is that exposure of the ovary to androgens leads to PCO, and certainly PCO is strongly associated with androgenic states; however, hard data on this are difficult to find, particularly on the transition from normal to polycystic structure.

A genetic cause for PCO

Several genes are probably implicated in the aetiology of PCO. The 21-hydroxylase gene is one candidate, and other clearly genetic conditions are associated with PCO.

A rare mutation of the insulin receptor gene causing resistance to signal transduction leads to gross hyperinsulinaemia of type A insulin resistance (IR), and all patients have PCOS. However, nearly all women with PCOS have normal insulin receptors. Few monogenic disorders are known, and the search is on for polygenes that contribute to the development of PCO.

Some evidence of genetic involvement in PCOS is that 85% of female relatives of an affected woman have PCO, and pedigrees show clear autosomal dominant inheritance with probably several contributing genes (2, 3, 4).

The environmental switch: the role of insulin

Several non-genetic factors may trigger the development of PCO in a female with a genetic disposition. PCO is clearly associated with obesity and high serum testosterone. In addition, insulin, acting as a co-gonadotrophin to luteinizing hormone (LH), is implicated in the development of PCO in adolescence, which is a time of physiological insulin resistance (IR). Hyperinsulinaemia is also found in many lean women with PCOS. Increased fat mass, obesity and hyperinsulinaemia are features of puberty (5).

The environmental switch: the role of leptin

An obvious candidate for a key role in the development of PCO is leptin, a neuropeptide hormone of the tumour necrosis factor group, controlled by insulin, affecting gonadotrophin secretion, and produced by fat cells. A greater fat mass means increased leptin production (6).

The role of leptin was first elucidated in obese mice (*ob/ob* genotype) which exhibit hypogonadotrophic hypogonadism. Mice infused intraperitoneally with leptin eat less and lose weight. In addition, levels of LH and follicle-stimulating hormone and the weight of the ovaries and uterus increased; evidently leptin stimulated the hypothalamus, resulting in restoration of fertility (7, 8).

Leptin and PCOS

PCOS is associated with disordered fat mass, insulin function and gonadotrophin secretion. Insulin controls the *ob* gene in fat tissue. Leptin, binding in the hypothalamus, having a direct connection with the GnRH neurone, and stimulating gonadotrophin secretion might provide a mechanism for a high serum LH level in PCOS.

Some other questions prompted us to study leptin levels in women with PCOS. For example, do androgens mediate the much lower leptin levels found in men than in women? What effect does IR have, and why does the ovary itself remain responsive to insulin? Figure 1 shows the relationship between (log) serum leptin level and body mass index in about 50 unselected patients with PCOS.

In this population about one-third of values fall below the normal range, these patients having lower leptin levels than their body mass index would predict. This is not yet explained, but there may be a mixture of inherited IR and the IR of puberty, together with under-reporting of weight increase; further weight gain then worsens IR, affecting leptin expression. It is interesting to note that leptin does not seem to affect androgen secretion, nor do androgens suppress leptin.

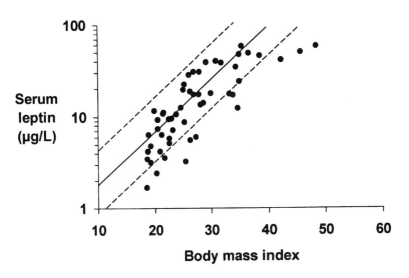

Fig. 1 Relationship between (log) serum leptin level and body mass index in about 50 unselected patients with PCOS.

Leptin and gonadotrophins in PCOS

We have found that leptin and gonadotrophin levels are correlated in women with PCOS (although the coefficient of correlation r for LH does not quite reach statistical significance):follicle-stimulating hormone, $r=0.35$ ($P=0.017$); LH, $r=0.26$ ($P=0.09$).

We do not yet understand interactions of leptin with the GnRH neurone, nor exactly how it stimulates the ovary to become polycystic (9).

Angiogenesis and PCO

Ultrasound measurements of ovarian volumes in PCO and in PCOS show that the total cyst volume is very small, but that the stroma is much enlarged. In addition, Doppler ultrasound demonstrates that blood flow through the stroma in both PCO and PCOS is roughly double that in normal controls (16 vs 8 cm/s).

It may be that ovarian angiogenesis precedes any endocrine change in PCO, and it has been found that serum levels of ubiquitous angiogenic factor vascular endothelial growth factor (VEGF) increase in normal ovaries during the preovulatory phase, rising still further in the luteal phase.

Thus VEGF is a serum marker for ovarian blood flow comparable with Doppler flow measurement. Preliminary data in 12 patients with PCO indicate that indeed VEGF levels did show an excess above that in normal ovaries, that paralleled the Doppler measurements (10, 11).

References

1   Bridges NA, Cooke A, Healy MJ, Hindmarsh PC & Brook CG. Ovaries in sexual precocity. *Clinical Endocrinology* 1995 **42** 135-140.

2   Bridges NA, Cooke A, Healy MJ, Hindmarsh PC & Brook CG. Standards for ovarian volume in childhood and puberty. *Fertility and Sterility* 1993 **60** 456-460.

3   Carey AH, Chan KL, Short F, White D, Williamson R & Franks S. Evidence for a single gene effect causing polycystic ovaries and male pattern baldness. *Clinical Endocrinology* 1993 **38** 653-658.

4   Franks S. Polycystic ovary syndrome: a changing perspective. *Clinical Endocrinology* 1989 **31** 87-120.

5   Smith CP, Archibald HR, Thomas JM, Tarn AC, Williams AJK, Gale EAM & Savage MO. Basal and stimulated insulin levels rise with advancing puberty. *Clinical Endocrinology* 1988 **28** 7-14.

6   Considine RV, Sinha MK, Heiman ML *et al*. Serum-immunoreactive leptin concentrations in normal-weight and obese humans. *New England Journal of Medicine* 1996 **334** 292-5.

7   Chehab FF, Lim ME & Lu R. Correction of the sterility defect in homozygous obese female mice by treatment with the human recombinant leptin. *Nature Genetics* 1996 **12** 318-320.

8   Barash IA, Cheung CC & Weigle DS. Leptin is a metabolic signal to the reproductive system. *Endocrinology* 1996 **137** 3144-3147.

9   Conway GS & Jacobs HS. Leptin: a hormone of reproduction. *Human Reproduction* 1997 **12** 633-635.

10   Zaidi J, Barber J, Kyei Mensah A, Bekir J, Campbell S & Tan SL. Relationship of ovarian stromal blood flow at the baseline ultrasound scan to subsequent follicular response in an in vitro fertilization program. *Obstetrics and Gynecology* 1996 **88** 779-84.

11   Agrawal R, Chimusoro K, Payne N, van der Spuy Z & Jacobs HS. *Current Opinion in Obstetrics and Gynecology* 1997 **9** 141-144.

Weight- and exercise-related endocrine disorders

Adolescent Endocrinology
Ed R Stanhope
BioScientifica Ltd, Bristol (1998)

The control of fat mass: insights from mouse genetics

S O'Rahilly and S Farooqi

Departments of Medicine and Clinical Biochemistry, University of Cambridge, Addenbrooke's Hospital, Cambridge, UK

The existence in mammals of signalling mechanisms controlling body weight in general and fat mass in particular has long been postulated, but little information on the molecular basis of any homoeostatic control mechanism has been available. Since 1994, however, no less than five different monogenic mouse models of obesity have been cloned and characterized (Table 1) (1-5). These studies have provided unique insights into the mechanisms that control energy expenditure and nutrient partitioning and the possible role of single gene defects in human obesity is currently the focus of intensive research.

Table 1 Summary of single gene defects in mouse models of obesity

Mouse gene	Chromosomal location	Nature of defect
ob	6	Mutation in coding region of leptin gene
db	4	Mutation in hypothalamic form of leptin receptor
fat	7	Defective carboxypepitdase E leading to impaired prohormone processing
tub	2	Mutation in a phosphodiesterase - like molecule expressed in the hypothalmus
agouti	8	Melanocortin 4 receptor antagonist

Leptin: the key to murine obesity syndromes

Discovery of leptin

Work on the genetics of obesity began 40 years ago, when the mouse *ob/ob* recessive syndrome of severe obesity, diabetes and infertility was first described by Ingalls *et al.* (6) The next obesity syndrome to be discovered was *db/db*, very similar to *ob/ob* (7). The experiments of Coleman and colleagues in the USA on parabiosis between *ob/ob* and *db/db* mice provided the key to these syndromes (8):

- normal + *db/db* - the normal mouse stopped eating and died of starvation;
- normal + *ob/ob* - the *ob/ob* mouse lost some fat;
- *ob/ob* + *db/db* - the *ob/ob* mouse stopped eating and died from starvation.

These experiments demonstrated that the *db/db* mouse was insensitive to a satiety factor circulating at high levels in its bloodstream, and that the *ob/ob* mouse lacked this factor.

It was not until 1994 that Freidman and colleagues (1) finally identified the gene for the satiety factor, which they named leptin. Leptin was not, as expected, produced in the brain, but was shown to be a peptide hormone secreted by the fat cells (adipocytes) of most vertebrates. A stop codon was found in the DNA of the leptin-deficient *ob/ob* mouse, preventing the leptin gene from being expressed.

Functions of leptin

Only 5 months after this work was published, three groups separately showed that leptin injected into *ob/ob* mice normalized not only their appetite and body weight but also their low body temperature and energy expenditure (9-11). Serum insulin and serum glucose were also normalized in the *ob/ob* mice; leptin had effectively cured their diabetes. Furthermore, leptin in sufficient quantity had the same effects in normal as in *ob/ob* mice, and the homologous human peptide was as effective as the murine peptide.

Mode of action of leptin

Leptin was much more potent when injected into the cerebrospinal fluid than intravenously, suggesting that it operates in the brain, and Tartaglia's group discovered that radiolabelled leptin bound to a receptor in the choroid plexus which closely resembled the GP-130 interleukin receptor (12). Confusingly, this putative leptin receptor was also found in the hypothalamus, lung, liver, kidney and skeletal muscle.

The simultaneous cloning of the defect in the leptin-resistant (receptor-defective) *db/db* mouse, by Tartaglia's, Friedman's and Leibel's groups (2, 13, 14) has resolved this confusion. Five or more alternatively spliced versions of the receptor exist, and in the *db* mouse an aberrant splicing event results in the removal of the intracellular signalling component of the receptor version that is highly expressed only in the hypothalamus.

Leptin in humans

Expression of the ob gene

Overexpression of leptin in the adipocytes of obese humans has been demonstrated by *in vitro* hybridization (15). Omental fat cells from grossly obese humans, particularly women, express more leptin mRNA than normals, and the degree of overexpression is correlated with the body mass index (BMI) (16).

Circulating leptin levels

Plasma leptin levels correlate with obesity in humans (17), but this does not imply, as has often been assumed, that leptin resistance is the only phenomenon linked to obesity; the relative contributions of resistance and deficiency to the high leptin levels in obesity are not yet understood. Dietary weight loss is accompanied by decreases in serum leptin and leptin mRNA in subcutaneous fat.

Neuroendocrine and reproductive functions of leptin

Apart from its role in the control of appetite and body weight, leptin has neuroendocrine and reproductive functions. Fasting in mice induced delayed vaginal oestrus, and abnormalities in testosterone, thyroxine and corticosteroid which were partially or completely normalized by treatment with leptin (18). Such interactions may be related to the amenorrhoea of anorexia nervosa and starvation.

Leptin and patterns of obesity

We have studied the differences between mRNA levels in subcutaneous fat and omental fat (responsible for central obesity) in 24 normal and moderately obese subjects (19). We have found that subcutaneous adipocytes significantly overexpress leptin mRNA relative to those in the omentum ($P<0.0001$). This difference is most dramatic in females (5.5±1.1-fold vs 1.9±0.2-fold in males). BMI correlates strongly with subcutaneous, but not with omental, leptin mRNA levels ($r=0.69$, $P<0.006$) in females, but no correlation is seen in males. Females store most fat in the subcutaneous depot, whilst in males storage tends to be more intra-abdominal. This sexually determined pattern of fat distribution may explain the well-established sexual dimorphism in plasma leptin levels.

A teleological explanation for why omental fat produces relatively little leptin could be that it has a very fast turnover, and long ago when man was subjected to attack by predators and to an uncertain food supply, it may once have been more appropriate to lay down reserves in an easily accessible depot than to control appetite. One could also speculate along these lines on explanations for differences between the sexes.

The *fat/fat* mouse

Another murine obesity syndrome is the *fat/fat* mouse. *Fat/fat* mice develop less extreme obesity, and develop it later in life, than *ob/ob* mice. Hyperglucocorticoidism seems not to be a feature, and only a small proportion (all of them males) have diabetes. Unlike all the other known murine obesity syndromes, however, they are extremely sensitive to injected insulin, even though they at first appeared already to have very high serum insulin levels. In fact these mice are not hyperinsulinaemic, but hyperproinsulinaemic, a condition caused by a mutation in the gene for carboxypeptidase E, a key enzyme in the transformation of proinsulin to insulin.

An implication for humans?

A woman referred to our clinic had had severe childhood obesity and lifelong symptoms of fatigue and low blood glucose levels between meals. A prolonged oral glucose tolerance test and high-performance liquid chromatography showed that she had high serum levels of intact and des-64, 65-proinsulin, but no detectable insulin. The proinsulin gene in this patient is normal, and the defect appears to be a heterozygous missense mutation in the gene for prohormone convertase-1 (PC-1) enzyme (20).

So, in the mouse world at least, the adipocyte has progressed during the last 2 or 3 years from a boring inert piece of lard to an extremely exciting active participant in the endocrine axis. The full therapeutic impact of these new findings on humans remains to be demonstrated.

References

1   Zhang Y, Proenca R, Maffei M, Barone M, Leopold L, Friedman JM, Naggert JK, Fricker LD, Varlamov O, Nishina PM, Rouille Y, Steiner DF, Carroll RJ, Paigen BJ & Leiter EH. Positional cloning of the mouse obese gene and its human homologue. *Nature* 1994 **372** 425-432.

2   Lee GH, Proenca R, Montez JM, Carroll KM, Darvishzadeh JG, Lee JI & Friedman JM. Abnormal splicing of the leptin receptor in diabetic mice. *Nature* 1996 **379** 632-635.

3   Huszar D, Lynch CA, Fairchild-Huntress V, Dunmore JH, Fang Q, Berkemeier LR, Gu W, Kesterson RA, Boston BA, Cone RD, Smith FJ, Campfield LA, Burn P & Lee F. Targeted disruption of the melanocortin-4 receptor results in obesity in mice. *Cell* 1997 **88** 131-141.

4   Naggert JK, Fricker LD, Varlamov O, Nishina PM, Rouille Y, Steiner DF, Carroll RJ, Paigen BJ & Leiter EH. Hyperproinsulinaemia in the obese fat/fat mice associated with a carboxypeptidase E mutation which reduces enzyme activity. *Nature Genetics* 1995 **10** 135-142.

5   Kleyn PW, Fan W, Kovats SG, Lee JJ, Pulido JC, Wu Y, Berkemeier LR, Misumi DJ, Holmgren L, Charlat O, Woolf EA, Tayber O, Brody T, Shu P, Hawkins F, Kennedy B, Baldini L, Ebeling C, Alperin GD, Deeds J, Lakey ND, Culpepper J, Chen H, Glucksmann-Kuis MA, Moore KJ, *et al*. Identification and characterization of the mouse obesity gene Tubby: a member of the novel gene family. *Cell* 1996 **85** 281-290.

6   Ingalls AM, Dickie MM & Snell GD. Obese, new mutation in house mouse. *Journal of Heredity* 1950 **41** 317-318.

7   Hummel KP & Dickie MM & Coleman DL. Diabetes, a new mutation in the mouse. *Science* 1966 **153** 1127-1128.

8   Coleman DL. Effects of parabiosis of obese with diabetes and normal mice. *Diabetologica* 1973 **9** 294-298.

9   Pelleymounter MA, Cullen MJ, Baker MB, Hecht R, Winters D, Boone T & Collins F. Effects of the obese gene product on body weight regulation in *ob/ob* mice. *Science* 1995 **269** 540-543.

10   Halaas JL, Gajiwala KS, Maffei M, Cohen SL, Chait BT, Rabinowitz D, Lallone RL, Burley SK & Friedman JM. Weight-reducing effects of the plasm protein encoded by the obese gene. *Science* 1995 **269** 543-546.

11   Campfield LA, Smith FJ, Guisez Y, Devos R & Burn P. Recombinant mouse Ob protein: evidence for a peripheral signal linking adiposity and central neural networks. *Science* 1995 **269** 546-549.

12   Devos R, Richards JG, Campfield LA, Tartaglia LA, Guisez Y, van der Heyden J, Travernier J, Plaetinck G & Burn P. Ob protein binds specifically to the choroid plexus of mice and rats. *Proceedings of the National Academy of Sciences of the USA* 1996 **93** 14795-14799.

13   Chen H, Charlat O, Tartaglia LA, Woolf EA, Weng X, Ellis SJ, Lakey ND, Culpepper J, Moore KJ, Breitbart RE, Duyk GM, Tepper RI & Morgenstem JP. Evidence that the diabetes gene encodes the leptin receptor: identification of a mutation in the leptin receptor gene in *db/db* mice. *Cell* 1996 **84** 491-495.

14   Chua SC Jr, Chung WK, Wu-Peng XS, Zhang Y, Liu SM, Tartaglia L & Leibel RL. Phenotypes of mouse diabetes and rat fatty due to mutations in the Ob (leptin) receptor. *Science* 1996 **271** 994-996.

15   Maffei M, Halaas J, Ravussin E, Pratley RE, Lee GH, Zhang Y, Fei H, Kim S, Lallone R, Ranganathan S, *et al.* Leptin levels in human and rodent, measurement of plasma leptin and *ob* RNA in obese and weight-reduced subjects. *Nature Medicine* 1995 **1** 1155-1161.

16   Hamilton BS, Paglia D, Kwan AY & Deitel M. Increased obese mRNA expression in omental fat cells from massively obese humans. *Nature Medicine* 1995 **1** 953-956.

17   Considine RV, Sinha MK, Heiman ML, Kriauciunas A, Stephens TW, Nyce MR, Ohannesian JP, Marco CC, McKee LJ, Bauer TL, *et al.* Serum immunoreactive leptin concentrations in normal-weight and obese humans. *New England Journal of Medicine* 1996 **334** 292-295.

18   Ahima RS, Prabakaran D, Mantzoros C, Qu D, Lowell B, Maratos-Flier E & Flier JS. Role of leptin in the neuroendocrine response to fasting. *Nature* 1996 **382** 250-252.

19   Montague CT, Prins JB, Sanders L, Digby JE & O'Rahilly S. Depot and sex-specific differences in human leptin mRNA expression: implications for the control of regional fat distribution. *Diabetes* 1997 **46** 342-347.

20   O'Rahilly S, Gray H, Humphreys PJ, Krook A, Polonsky KS, White A, Gibson S, Taylor K & Carr C. Brief report: impaired processing of prohormones associated with abnormalities of glucose homeostasis and adrenal function. *New England Journal of Medicine* 1995 **333** 1386-1390.

Adolescent Endocrinology
Ed R Stanhope
BioScientifica Ltd, Bristol (1998)

Weight and reproductive endocrine dysfunction

S Franks

Department of Obstetrics and Gynaecology, Imperial School of
Medicine at St Mary's, London, UK

The common theme in the relationship between body weight and ovarian function in puberty and adolescence, and in states of under- and over-nutrition is an excess or deficiency of insulin. Insulin may mediate the effects of nutritional alterations on the hypothalamic-pituitary-gonadal axis.

Ovarian function and body weight

Leptin, insulin, body weight and ovarian function

It is well known that obesity may advance puberty and menarche, while being underweight may delay these events. It has been postulated that a signal passes from fat cells to the hypothalamus and so controls gonadotrophin secretion. Leptin is a likely candidate, particularly as its expression is mediated by insulin.

The following questions arise: (1) does leptin mediate changes in the hypothalamic-pituitary-ovarian axis during normal developmental disorders of ovarian function? (2) is leptin deficiency the cause of amenorrhoea in anorexia? and (3) does leptin play a role in obesity and polycystic ovary syndrome (PCOS)? Dr G S Conway has shown in this volume that leptin levels and the secretion of gonadotrophin-releasing hormone are correlated, and that neuropeptide-Y probably plays a part in this relationship. Patients with PCOS in Dr Conway's series show an abnormal relationship between leptin levels and body mass index (BMI). Further work is needed to clarify these areas, and it is not yet known whether leptin deficiency (or excess) or leptin receptor abnormalities have a role in subgroups of women with PCOS. Leptin may be only one of several cytokines produced by fat cells acting as metabolic signals and affecting hypothalamic function.

Insulin may, however, have a direct bearing on gonadal function during puberty. Insulin levels change during puberty and adolescence and, as Dr Conway also noted, insulin acts as a co-gonadotrophin. It may therefore have a role as a co-ordinator of growth and reproductive function.

As shown by Holly and colleagues (1), insulin levels rise during adolescence; this is related, particularly in girls, to increased fat and fat distribution. Levels of sex-hormone-binding globulin (SHBG) follow those of insulin, and are associated with increased concentrations of free oestradiol and testosterone. Changes in insulin-like growth factor-binding protein-1 also occur, but it is not yet known whether they affect levels of circulating insulin-like growth factor-I. These findings add further weight to the hypothesis that insulin is a nutritional signal that co-ordinates both growth and reproductive function.

Undernutrition and ovarian function

Weight loss is one of the most common causes of disordered reproductive function; among a series of 73 consecutive patients studied in our own clinic, 27 (38%) had amenorrhoea related to weight loss. The influence of undernutrition on gonadotrophin secretion is primarily at the hypothalamic rather than pituitary level.

Obesity, ovarian function and PCOS

Obesity and infertility

One of the earliest references to the effects of obesity on fertility can be found in the writings of Hippocrates. He describes the Scythians as follows.

'The girls get amazingly flabby and podgy. People of such constitution cannot be prolific. Fatness and flabbiness are to blame. The womb is unable to receive the semen, and they menstruate infrequently and little. The opening of the womb is sealed by fat and does not permit insemination.'

'As good proof of the sort of physical characteristics that are favourable to conception, consider the case of serving-wenches: no sooner do they have intercourse with a man than they become pregnant, on account of their sturdy physique and their leanness of flesh.' (2)

Some more recent studies have also drawn attention to the relationship between obesity, infertility and menstrual disturbance (3-6), although none of these has focused on the importance of possible differences between women with normal ovaries and those with polycystic ovaries.

Insulin and PCOS

PCOS is associated with hyperinsulinaemia and insulin resistance (7-9). Even in lean women with PCOS, insulin sensitivity is lower than in weight-matched controls. It is further reduced in obese subjects compared with weight-matched controls.

Recent studies from Holte and colleagues have advanced our understanding of the relationship between PCOS, insulin insensitivity and obesity (8). Insulin sensitivity declines significantly with increasing BMI in control subjects; but in those with PCOS the slope of the regression line is significantly steeper than that of controls. Thus, BMI and polycystic ovaries interact in the determination of insulin sensitivity.

Metabolic changes associated with polycystic ovaries differ according to menstrual cyclicity. Women who have polycystic ovaries and regular cycles have slightly elevated luteinizing hormone (LH) levels, which are intermediate between those of women with the classic syndrome of anovulatory PCOS with hyperandrogenism and those of controls. Testosterone levels in women who have polycystic ovaries and regular cycles are similar to those in the classic syndrome, but their metabolic profile is clearly different (10).

Insulin sensitivity is lower in women with classic PCOS than in weight-matched lean or obese controls. Insulin sensitivity in equally hyperandrogenaemic women with regular cycles is, however, not significantly diminished (9). Plasma insulin concentration after an oral glucose load shows a comparable disparity between these two groups; stimulated insulin levels are much higher in women with oligomenorrhoea than in controls, but close to normal in weight-matched subjects with regular cycles.

This relationship between insulin sensitivity, insulin levels and menstrual cyclicity suggests that raised insulin levels, decreased insulin sensitivity, or both, may be involved in the mechanism of anovulation (11).

Effect of weight loss on ovarian function
Kiddy and colleagues (12) studied the effect of weight loss on ovarian function in 24 obese women with PCOS (mean weight about 90 kg), who received a 1000 kcal/day low-fat diet for 6 months. Relative to the remaining 11 subjects, the 13 with 'reasonable' weight loss (>5% of initial body weight) showed:
- a significant reduction in fasting and glucose-stimulated insulin levels
- a consequent rise in SHBG
- improved cyclicity, including five pregnancies among seven previously infertile women.

Similar reciprocal changes in fasting insulin and SHBG were also seen in obese control subjects who lost weight, but they are likely to be more significant in women with PCOS, who are hyperandrogenaemic and relatively more hyperinsulinaemic and insulin resistant.

Hyperinsulinaemia, insulin resistance and anovulation

How are hyperinsulinaemia and insulin resistance related to the mechanism of anovulation? Studies in our department have shown that, in women with PCOS and peripheral insulin resistance, ovarian granulosa cells remain responsive to insulin (13); insulin resistance therefore appears to be tissue-specific.

Arrested follicular development: action of LH and insulin on granulosa cells
In anovulatory women with PCOS, follicular development is arrested at about 5-8 mm diameter. Excess secretion of LH and insulin may be the key factors contributing to this arrest.

LH has differential effects on steroidogenesis and growth in the maturing follicle, mediated by intracellular cAMP; the higher the level of cAMP, the greater the likelihood of terminal differentiation and arrested growth (11). However, arrest of growth with maintained steroidogenesis is normal after onset of the LH surge. It has recently been confirmed in our department that

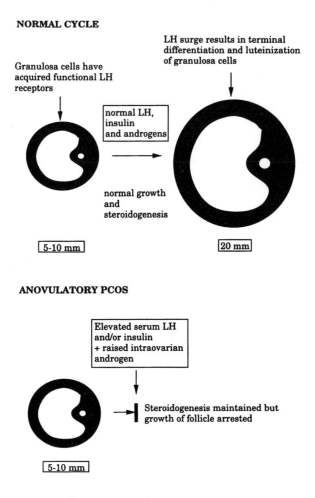

Fig. 1 Proposed mechanism for anovulation in PCOS. In the normal cycle, granulosa cells acquire functional LH receptors when the follicle is about 10 mm in diameter. Growth and steroidogenesis are maintained by FSH and low levels of LH in the face of normal insulin and androgen concentrations. Terminal differentiation/luteinization is triggered by the onset of the LH surge. In anovulatory PCOS, elevated serum concentrations of LH and/or insulin, together with raised intrafollicular androgens, may combine to promote premature luteinization and arrest of follicle growth. Adapted with permission from (11).

LH responsiveness occurs in granulosa cells at the 10 mm follicular diameter stage, so that in the late follicular stage they respond to both follicle-stimulating hormone (FSH) and LH. By contrast, it appears that, in anovulatory women with polycystic ovaries, even the smaller follicles (3-4 mm diameter) respond to LH (14).

Could elevated serum LH or increased responsiveness to LH affect follicular maturation? We have found that insulin profoundly affects the response of granulosa cells to LH *in vitro*. Cells preincubated with FSH, which is involved in the acquisition of LH receptors, increase oestradiol production in response to LH alone, but this response is enormously and synergistically increased when insulin is present in the preincubation medium (13). In subjects with PCOS this phenomenon might lead to anovulation in the following way. When a follicle has reached 10 mm diameter, raised LH levels (or more probably elevated insulin levels interacting with raised LH) cause increased steroidogenesis; but elevated LH levels (or increased responsiveness to LH) may also lead to premature arrest of follicle growth because the net LH signal at this stage is as great as that normally found only in the preovulatory phase at the beginning of the LH surge (Fig. 1).

Summary

Weight gain and changing body fat distribution during puberty are associated with maturation of the hypothalamic-pituitary-ovarian axis. Insulin, and perhaps leptin, may be important nutritionally triggered signals in this process. Undernutrition resulting in weight loss reverses the normal maturational changes in the hypothalamic-pituitary-ovarian axis, and it is tempting to think that leptin or other cytokines produced by fat cells may mediate the observed hypothalamic changes. Obesity causes hyperinsulinaemia, particularly in PCOS, where the polycystic ovary interacts with BMI. In addition, insulin may have a direct adverse effect on follicular maturation that is particularly relevant to the mechanism of anovulation in women with PCOS.

References

1   Holly JMP, Smith CP, Dunger DB, Howell RJ, Chard T, Perry LA, Savage MO, Cianfarani S, Rees LH & Wass JA. Relationship between the fall in sex hormone-binding globulin and insulin-like growth factor binding protein-I. A synchronized approach to pubertal development. *Clinical Endocrinology* 1989 **31** 277-284.

2   Hippocrates. Airs, waters, places (an essay on the influences of climate, water supply and situation on health). In: *Hippocratic Writings*, pp 164-165. Eds J Chadwick & WN Mann. London: Penguin, 1978.

3   Hartz AJ, Barboriak PN, Wong A, Katayama KP & Rimm AA. The association of obesity with infertility and related menstrual abnormalities in women. *International Journal of Obesity* 1979 **3** 57-73.

4   Kopelmann PG, Pilkington TRE, White N & Jeffcoate SL. The effect of weight loss on sex steroid secretion and binding in massively obese women. *Clinical Endocrinology* 1981 **14** 113-116.

5   Harlass FE, Plymate SR, Farris BL & Belts RP. Weight loss associated with correction of gonadotropin and sex steroid abnormalities in the obese anovulatory female. *Fertility and Sterility* 1984 **42** 649-652.

6   Kiddy DS, Sharp PS, White DM, Scanlon MF, Mason HD, Bray CS, Polson DW, Reed MJ & Franks S. Differences in clinical and endocrine features between obese and non-obese subjects with polycystic ovary syndrome: an analysis of 263 consecutive cases. *Clinical Endocrinology* 1990 **32** 213-220.

7   Dunaif A. Insulin resistance and ovarian dysfunction. In: *Insulin Resistance*, pp 301-325. D Moller. New York: John Wiley, 1993.

8   Holte J. Disturbances in insulin secretion and sensitivity in women with the polycystic ovary syndrome. *Baillière's Clinical Endocrinology and Metabolism* 1996 **10** 221-247.

9   Robinson S, Kiddy D, Gelding SV, Willis D, Niththyananthan R, Bush A, Johnston DG & Franks S. The relationship of insulin sensitivity to menstrual pattern in women with hyperandrogenism and polycystic ovaries. *Clinical Endocrinology* 1993 **39** 351-355.

10   Franks S. Polycystic ovary syndrome: a changing perspective. *Clinical Endocrinology* 1989 **31** 87-120.

11   Franks S, Robinson S & Willis D. Nutrition, insulin and polycystic ovary syndrome. *Reviews of Reproduction* 1996 **1** 47-53.

12   Kiddy DS, Hamilton-Fairley D, Bush A, Short F, Anyaoku V, Reed MJ & Franks S. Improvement in endocrine and ovarian function during dietary treatment of obese women with polycystic ovary syndrome. *Clinical Endocrinology* 1992 **36** 105-111.

13   Willis D, Mason H, Gilling-Smith C & Franks S. Modulation by insulin of follicle stimulating and luteinizing hormone action in human granulosa cells of normal and polycystic ovaries. *Journal of Clinical Endocrinology and Metabolism* 1996 **81** 302-309.

14   Willis DS, Mason HD, Watson H, Galea R, Bricat M & Frank S. Characterization ofthe LH response in granulosa cells from individual follicles from normal and polycystic ovaries. *Programme of the 10th International Congress of Endocrinology, San Francisco* 1996 Abstract OR26-1.

Adolescent Endocrinology
Ed R Stanhope
BioScientifica Ltd, Bristol (1998)

Anabolic steroid and associated drug misuse

A R W Forrest

Department of Clinical Chemistry and Toxicology, Royal Hallamshire Hospital and Department of Forensic Pathology, University of Sheffield, Sheffield S10 2JF, UK

Adolescent males and others use a variety of drugs and other substances with the aim of achieving a physique that they perceive to be desirable. It is well known that anabolic steroids are often misused for this purpose, but so are many other types of drug: metabolic stimulants, modulators of the effects of anabolic steroids, post-exercise anabolism promoters, and even nutritional supplements. The list includes ephedrine, salicylates, zopiclone, γ-hydroxybutyrate, injectable analgesics, aminogluthemide and a host of others. The scientific basis for using many of them is questionable, to say the least. This chapter reviews their use among the body-building community, how to detect them, and the 'grey market' in which they are bought and sold.

Anabolic steroids

Table 1 shows just a few of the many anabolic steroids currently available. They come from all over the world, and many of them are not quite what they claim to be.

Table 1 Some of the many anabolic steroids currently available to body builders on the 'grey market'

Fluoxymesterone	Oxandrolone
Methandienone	Oxymetholone
Methandrostenolone	Stanozolol
Methanolone	Testosterone
Nandrolone	Trenbolone

Organized crime is moving into the area of anabolic steroids and has the resources to produce counterfeit products complete with packaging, labelling, and even ceramic-printed ampoules. In our laboratory we have seen anabolic steroids originating in Thailand, Greece, South America, Kenya, India and

Pakistan; Eastern European products, from Bulgaria and elsewhere, are generally of good quality. However, there is a considerable amount of 'snipe' or counterfeit material available. About 40% of the samples examined in our laboratory contain an anabolic steroid other than that specified on the package label. About 10% contain no identifiable anabolic steroid. *Caveat emptor* with a vengeance.

Growth promoters/hormones

Some drugs coming into use that are of particular interest to endocrinologists are insulin-like growth factor-I, growth hormone and insulin. Growth hormone circulating among the body-building community in particular has not been kept in the cold chain (ie refrigerated from manufacture to point of use), and is of very poor quality by the time it reaches the end user, although this may change as new products appear that do not need refrigeration. At least some of the growth hormone on the grey market is of human pituitary material not recombinant material. Insulin is another drug used after exercise in a low dose (5-10 U) in the belief that it potentiates the anabolic response. The use of insulin in this context is a good example of the way in which body builders may take good research and apply it inappropriately and out of context.

Legal highs, smart drugs and supplements

The marketing and use of anabolic steroids have recently become linked to those of so-called legal highs, smart drugs and nutritional supplements. Legal highs include stimulants such as caffeine, ephedrine and kava (*Piper methysticum*); some smart drugs are also stimulants, including neurotransmitter precursors such as procaine, a precursor of acetylcholine and a component of the notorious 'antigeriatric agent' KH 19 that was reputed to sustain some former Eastern Bloc heads of state into extreme age. The term smart drugs also embraces extracts of banana and many other agents.

All these products are marketed in a 'grey' semi-legal area; some merchants who tablet up vitamin supplements might move into legal highs, smart drugs and, perhaps, controlled drugs. (At this point, hopefully, they attract the attention of law enforcement agencies.) In the UK the enforcement agencies are now taking a more proactive approach to the control of products containing ephedrine. Consequently, there has been a resurgence in the market for unlicensed products containing large amounts of caffeine. While these may be used as 'fat burners' by body builders, they are more commonly encountered as 'dance drugs'. Many formulations are embossed with symbols similar to those that appear on ecstasy tablets, such as a '£' sign or the 'White Tornado' logo.

Diagnosing steroid misuse

This paper does not address the specialized field of drug misuse in sports medicine (1). The clinical endocrinologist typically sees individuals who have been referred after abusing anabolic steroids, encountering problems, and consulting their primary care physician. A patient who does not admit to what he is using is best approached by way of a urine steroid profile, looking for unusual peaks of exogenous anabolic steroids or their metabolites, an unusual profile (e.g. high or low androgen levels and/or high or low androgen/cortisol ratio, and high creatinine) (2). In practice, a good primary screen is the ratio of total androgens to total cortisol metabolites; if this is abnormal, further derivatization and extraction steps will identify the anabolic steroids concerned, although this is seldom necessary.

Not only anabolic steroids...

Apart from anabolic supplements, users of all ages employ nutritional supplements and metabolic modulators, sometimes with encouragement from pharmaceutical companies, together with a generous dose of 'magical thinking'. The commonest piece of magical thinking is: 'More Is Always Better'.

The use of these compounds may be based on: good science with a clear rationale; research findings taken out of context (the newly recognized hormone leptin, or compounds purporting to be leptin, will surely appear soon on the grey market); rumour and custom (often as promulgated by the trainers); or no obvious rationale whatsoever.

Table 2 summarizes the main classes of compound other than anabolic steroids used by body builders.

Table 2 Main classes of compound other than anabolic steroids used by body builders

Class	Examples
Metabolic stimulants	Caffeine, ephedrine, 'narnigens', β-agonists, thyroid hormones
Modulators of anabolic steroid effects	Antioestrogens, 5α-reductase inhibitors, acne treatments, hepatoprotective agents, human choriogonadotrophin
Post-exercise anabolism promoters	Nalbuphine, melatonin, γ-hydroxybutyrate, zopiclone, valproate
Nutritional supplements	Creatine, l-carnitine, arginine, aspartate, ornithine α-ketoglutarate, vanadium

Metabolic stimulants

Caffeine is freely available, and is in very common use, increasingly in forms containing much higher amounts than those found in tea or coffee. They include Jolt Cola, Red Bull (a smart drug that also contains metabolic precursors) and guarana (a stimulant used by the Amazonian Indians). Caffeine is also widely used in combination products.

Ephedrine is now being controlled more tightly in the UK and its illegal marketing cut down. It has largely disappeared from the open shelves of the purveyors of legal highs in the UK, although it can still be purchased in gymnasia. The rationale for its use is that it helps burn off body fat in preparation for a competition. It appears in Chinese medicines such as Ma Huang, and in the original version of the product Ultimate Orange. Ultimate Orange is a nutritional supplement containing sugars plus large amounts of ephedrine and caffeine. Ephedrine is also taken in simple powder form (sometimes by the spoonful), and some users progress from this to street amphetamines.

'Narnigens' are grapefruit flavenoids alleged to promote fat mobilization. They are often found as poorly made tablets also containing ephedrine, aspirin and caffeine, and are promoted as 'fat-burners'.

Of the β-agonists, clenbuterol often enters the UK mainly from Spain, legally carried through customs by users who declare it for their own personal use (often bringing in as much as they can carry – and they can carry a lot). Salbutamol does not have the same anabolic effects as clenbuterol, but there is anecdotal evidence that it has been misused in an amphetamine-like way, being obtained from general practitioners for 'asthma' and taken in large amounts by body builders; dangerous hypokalaemia is a possible consequence of this practice.

Thyroid hormones, usually tri-iodothyronine, are taken by body builders to burn off weight before a competition.

Modulators of anabolic steroid effects

Substances that can modulate some of the undesired effects of anabolic steroids are also widely used.

Antioestrogens are common particularly when testosterones are used. Tamoxifen is used, together with other oestrogen antagonists not available in the UK such as toramifene. Aminoglutethemide (Orimeten) and other aromatase inhibitors may be used. The purpose of antioestrogen and aromatase inhibitor use is to prevent the development of hyperpigmentation of the nipples and gynaecomastia ('Witches teat').

5α-Reductase inhibitors including finasteride (Proscar) are used by male users of anabolic steroids for prostatic symptoms such as nocturia, which they commonly encounter.

Acne, particularly on the back, is very common in anabolic steroid users, and is not acceptable in competitive body builders. Therefore acne treatments are used. A worrying development is the appearance of anti-acne isoretinoic acid derivatives (isotretinoin-Roaccutane) among the illegal drug using community; a particular danger is that these teratogenic drugs may be passed to female users who are at risk of pregnancy.

Hepatoprotective agents are also taken. Silmarin (Legalon) is a derivative of the milk thistle *Silybum marianum* legally available in several European countries. It is used clinically to promote biliary secretion, and extracts have long been used as a folk remedy for dry cows. It has also been used experimentally with the aim of countering hepatotoxicity associated with Amanita mushroom poisoning, and individuals using potentially hepatoxic 17α anabolic steroids may take it for the alleged hepatoprotective effect.

Human chorionic gonadotrophin is commonly taken at the end of a cycle of anabolic steroids to restore testicular function.

Post-exercise anabolism promoters

Nalbuphine (Nubain) is one of the less well-known drugs used by body builders in the UK with the aim of encouraging anabolism after exercise. This injectable opiate is not a controlled substance, but tolerance and withdrawal syndromes do occur and I know of two users who went on to use street heroin. It may also be used before martial arts exhibition bouts or displays as a pre-emptive analgesic.

Melatonin, γ-hydroxy-butyrate (GHB), zopiclone and valproate (Epilim) are all available in the UK. GHB is easy to synthesize, recipes being available that require little knowledge of chemistry and only the equipment found in the average kitchen. All may be taken with the objective of extending the post-exercise anabolic window. GHB has also been used as a disco drug, as it induces mild intoxication. Zopiclone is a non-benzodiazepine hypnotic, and one illicit route of importation into the UK from France has been mail-order via the Irish Republic. Some non-controlled substances are also being obtained by mail order through the Internet.

Nutritional supplements

Creatine, l-carnitine, vitamin B, arginine, aspartate, ornithine α-ketoglutarate and vanadium are among the many nutritional supplements promoted as aids to body building. The body's requirement for vanadium is minute, but this element is being taken in 7.5mg tablets, with effects that can only be guessed at. The 'Ultimate Nutritional Supplement' which I recently encountered purported to be an 'amino acid' supplement. The capsules also contained substantial amounts of the anabolic steroid Stanozolol. At least this was one product that would be effective.

Controlling bodies

In the UK, the availability of misused food and food additive substances is controlled by the Trading Standards Authority, medicines and substances promoted as producing a physiological effect in the user, rather than simple food additives, by the Medicines Control Agency, and controlled drugs by the police, under the Misuse of Drugs Act. The situation is complex; for example, caffeine may be regarded as a flavouring agent in, for example, cola drinks, and as a medicinal substance under the terms of the Medicine Act in products such as Pro-Plus.

Information sources for drug misusers

I suspect that much information about drugs and their misuse is being provided in 'sports science' courses, both at undergraduate and Master's level. To my own knowledge, people who supply anabolic steroids have enrolled on such courses in order to provide a better service to their clients. I believe it should be the stated policy of academic institutes that anyone caught dealing in such substances or advising on their use while taking a sports medicine or sports science course should be rusticated forthwith.

There are many sites on the world wide web that provide information about the topics discussed here; the quality of the web sites and mailing lists varies enormously. Much of the information provided is flawed and some is positively dangerous. There is also a considerable written literature available to the more literate user (3).

I acknowledge all the trade names quoted in this paper. The use of a trade name should not be taken as implying that the manufacturer of any product named or its legal distributors approve or in any way countenance the misuse of their products.

References

1   Bowers LD & Segura J. Anabolic steroids, athletic drug testing and the Olympic games. *Clinical Chemistry* 1996 **42** 999-1000.
2   Catlin DH, Hatton CK & Starcevic SH. Issues in detecting abuse of xenobiotic anabolic steroids and testosterone by analysis of athletes' urine. *Clinical Chemistry* 1997 **437** 1280-1288.
3   Duchaine D. *Underground Steroid Handbook Update.* Venice, CA: HLR Technica Books 1992.

Author index

Al-Shoumer K A S   17
Anyaoku V   17
Azziz R   79

Baird D   45
Beshyah S A   17

Chrisoulidou A   17
Conway G S   101

Davies M C   59

Farooqi S   107
Forrest A R W   119
Franks S   113

Huhtaniemi I   33

Ibáñez L   85

Jacobs H S   25
Johnston D G   17

Kousta E   17

O'Rahilly S   107

Parks J S   3
Porcu E   93
Potau N   85

Rees M   39

Seino Y   11

Vandeweghe M   51
Venturoli S   93

Zucker K J   71

Subject index

Page numbers in *italics* or **bold** indicate illustrations or tables appearing away from their text.

acne 80, 122
adrenal hypoplasia congenita (AHC), X-linked 4
adrenarche 85
    premature 85–91
adrenocorticotrophin (ACTH)
    in CAH 82
    stimulation test, in CAH 80–1
agouti **107**
alkaline phosphatase, serum bone (B-ALP) 13, 14
    GH therapy and 14–15
Alzheimer's disease
    age at menarche and 43
    effects of oestrogen 27–8
amenorrhoea
    primary
        in CAH 80
        in gonadotrophin receptor mutations 37
        osteoporosis 25–6
    treatment 59, *60*
    weight loss and 114
aminoglutethimide 122
anabolic steroids 119–20
    counterfeit 120
    diagnosing misuse 120–1
    information sources 124
    modulators of effects **121**, 122–3
anabolism promoters, post-exercise **121**, 123
androgens
    adrenal 85, *86*
        female foetus exposure 72, 74
        mechanisms of excess, in CAH 82–3
        in premature pubarche 85, *87*
    in anovulatory girls 93, *94*
    causing polycystic ovaries 101
    leptin and 103
    ovarian, in premature pubarche 89
androstenedione
    in anovulatory girls 93, *94*
    in premature pubarche 89
angiogenesis
    endometrial 41–2
    ovarian, in PCOS 103–4

anovulation 46
   in adolescence, PCOS development and 93–8
   mechanism in PCOS 115–17
   ovulation induction 47–9, 59
   see also polycystic ovary syndrome
antiandrogens, in CAH 83
antioestrogens
   misuse 122
   in PCOS 48, 59
aromatase inhibitors 122

birth order, age at menarche and 40
blood loss, menstrual 40–1
body builders, drug misuse 119–24
body composition, age at menarche and 39–40
bone
   formation in adolescence 12
   growth
      GH therapy and *15*, 16
      osteoporosis and 11–12
   growth rate (BGR) 12, *14*
   metabolic markers 13–14
      in adolescence 14
      effects of GH 14–15
bone mineral density (BMD)
   GH therapy and *15*, 16, 21
   HRT effects 26
   in oestrogen deficiency 25–6
   peak (PBM) 11
BRCA1 gene carriers 44
breast cancer
   age at menarche and 43
   HRT and 28–9
breast development, menarche and 43–4

caffeine 120, 121–2, 123–4
CAH *see* congenital adrenal hyperplasia
calcium supplementation 29
cancer
   age at menarche and 43
   fertility management after 64, 65, 66
   HRT risks 28–9
carboxypeptidase E gene mutation **107**, 110
cardiovascular disease
   age at menarche and 43
   in GH-deficient adults 17–18
   in GH-treated hypopituitary adults 20–1
   hyperinsulinaemia and 91
   in oestrogen deficiency 26–7
carotid artery disease, in GH-deficient adults 17–18
cerebrovascular disease, in GH-deficient adults 17

cholesterol, serum
    in GH-deficient adults 18, **19**
    in GH-treated hypopituitary adults 20
chromosomal anomalies, ICSI and 63, 64
chronic illness, age at menarche and 40
clenbuterol 122
cloning, positional 4
clotting, blood, in GH-deficient adults 20
collagen type I
    GH therapy and 15
    metabolism 14
    serum (P1CP) **13**, 14
collagen type I cross-linked C-telopeptide (1CTP) **13**, 14
collagen type I cross-linked N-telopeptide (1NTP) **13**, 14
colorectal cancer, age at menarche and 43
congenital adrenal hyperplasia (CAH) 72–4, 79–83
    carriers 81
    fertility treatment 62–3
    mechanisms of hyperandrogenism 82–3
    non-classical (NCAH, late-onset) 79–82, 85
        diagnosis 80–2
        genetics 79
    polycystic ovaries in 101
    psychosexual development in females 73–4
    salt-wasting (SW) 63, 79
        fertility 83
        psychosexual development 73–4
    simple virilizing (SV) 79
        fertility 83
        psychosexual development 73–4
    treatment of symptoms 83
contraception 42
coronary heart disease see ischaemic heart disease
costs, of CAH diagnosis 82
C-peptide, plasma, in GH-treated hypopituitary adults 20
cytochrome $P450c_{17\alpha}$ 85
    dysregulation 88, 89
    insulin action 90

Dax-1 gene 3, 4, 5
db/db mouse 107–8
dehydroepiandrosterone (DHEA), in premature pubarche 89–90
dehydroepiandrosterone sulphate (DHEAS)
    in non-classical CAH 80
    in premature pubarche 85, 87
depot contraceptives 42
diabetes mellitus, in GH-deficient adults 19–20
Doppler ultrasound, ovaries 101, 103–4
drug misuse 119–24
    agents other than anabolic steroids 121–3
    controlling bodies 123–4
    information sources 124
    see also anabolic steroids

endometrial cancer, HRT and 28
endometrium
    cell cultures 41, 42
    menstruation and 41–2
ephedrine 120, 122
exercise
    age at menarche and 40
    bone growth in adolescence and 12
    tolerance, GH therapy and 21

family size, age at menarche and 40
fat, body
    distribution
        in GH-deficient adults 18
        role of leptin 109
    mass, control 107–10
fat/fat mouse **107**, 109–10
fertility treatment 59–66
    in anovulation 47–9, 59–62
    in CAH 62–3
    in hypogonadotrophic hypogonadal males 54, 63
    in hypopituitary males 52, 53–4
finasteride 122
foetus
    female, virilization 72–3
    oocyte retrieval 65
follicles, ovarian
    arrested development, in PCOS 115–17
    development 34, 45
    maturation 34, *35*
    selection of dominant 47
follicle-stimulating hormone (FSH)
    action in developing ovary 35
    β-subunit mutation 4
    for ovulation induction 47, 48–9
    premature pubarche and 88, 89
    receptor mutation 36–7
    recombinant 47
    role in ovulation 45
folliculogenesis 34
fractures, osteoporotic 25–6
FSH *see* follicle-stimulating hormone

γ-hydroxy-butyrate (GHB) 123
gender identity/role 71
    in CAH 74
    conflicts 71–2
genetic factors
    in age at menarche 39
    in bone growth in adolescence 12
gestogens
    coronary heart disease and 27
    endometrial cancer and 28

GH *see* growth hormone
glucose tolerance
    in GH-deficient adults 19–20
    in GH-treated hypopituitary adults 20
    in premature pubarche 90–1
gonadotrophin-releasing hormone (GnRH, LHRH)
    analogues causing polycystic ovaries 95, 101
    gene mutations 3–4, 36
    pulsatile
        in hypogonadotrophic hypogonadal males 53–4
        in ovulation induction 48, 59, *61*
    receptor gene 3, *4*
    role in ovulation 45–6
    stimulation tests 88, 89–90
gonadotrophins
    action in developing ovary 35
    in anovulatory girls 93, *94*
    antagonists 49
    deficiency *see* hypogonadotrophic hypogonadism
    and leptin, in PCOS 103
    for ovulation induction 47–9
    receptor mutations 36–7
    recombinant 47, 49
    therapy 47–9
        complications 60–2
        hypogonadotrophic hypogonadal males 54
        hypopituitary males 53–4
    see also follicle-stimulating hormone (FSH); luteinizing hormone (LH)
growth hormone (GH)
    -deficient adults
        excess vascular disease 17–18
        mechanisms of vascular disease 18–20
        see also hypopituitarism
    misuse 120
    treatment
        causing polycystic ovaries 101
        effects on bone *15*, 16, 21
        metabolic bone markers and 14–15
        in young hypopituitary adults 17, 20–2
growth promoters/hormones 120

height
    hypopituitary males 52
    LH-β polymorphisms and 6
    in premature pubarche 86
Hippocrates 114
hirsutism 93, 98
    in CAH 80
    premature pubarche and 86, 88, 89
    treatment 83
hpg mouse 36
HRT *see* oestrogen/progesterone replacement therapy

human chorionic gonadotrophin (hCG)
    in hypogonadotrophic hypogonadal males 54
    in hypopituitary males 53–4
    misuse 123
Human Fertilization and Embryology Authority 66
human menopausal gonadotrophin (hMG)
    in hypogonadotrophic hypogonadal males 54
    in hypopituitary males 53–4
21-hydroxylase
    deficiency 72, 79, *80*
        carriers 81
    gene
        mutations 79
        polycystic ovaries and 102
17-hydroxyprogesterone (17-HP)
    in CAH 80–2
    in premature pubarche 89, 90
hyperandrogenism
    in anovulatory girls 93, 94, 97, 98
    functional ovarian *see* ovarian hyperandrogenism, functional
    hyperinsulinaemia as trigger 90
    mechanisms in CAH 82–3
hypergonadotrophic ovarian dysgenesis (HOD) 36–7
hyperinsulinaemia
    cardiovascular risk 91
    in PCOS 114–17
    in premature pubarche 90–1
    triggering hyperandrogenism 90
hyperproinsulinaemia, in *fat/fat* mice 110
hyp mouse 3–4
hypogonadotrophic hypogonadism (HH)
    adrenal hypoplasia congenita with 4
    causes 51
    combined with GH deficiency *see* hypopituitarism
    gene mutations 3–4
    male 51–5, 63
        acquired in adulthood 51
        GnRH vs. hCG/hMG therapy 54
        gonadotrophin therapy 54
        pulsatile LHRH therapy 54
    in *ob/ob* mice 102
    osteoporosis 25
    ovulation induction 48, 59, *61*
hypopituitarism 17–22
    GH therapy in young adults 17, 20–2
    male
        fertility induction 52, 53–4
        psychosexual adjustment 52, 53
        testosterone replacement therapy 52
    osteoporosis 25

vascular disease
    aetiologies 18–20
    excess mortality 17
    GH therapy and 21
    increased frequency 17–18
hypothalamic/pituitary/gonadal (HPG) axis
    body weight regulation and 113
    mutations affecting 3–5
    premature pubarche and 88

infertility 59–66
    in CAH 80, 83
    in gonadotrophin receptor mutations 37
    male 4, 63–4
    obesity and 114
    see also fertility treatment
information, for drug misusers 124
inhibin 46–7
insulin
    in aetiology of PCOS 102, 114–15
    in body weight control 113–14
    as co-gonadotrophin 102, 113
    in *fat/fat* mice 110
    granulosa cell responses in PCOS 115–17
    leptin interaction 102–3
    misuse 120
    receptor
        gene mutations 102
        serine phosphorylation 90
    resistance (IR)
        in PCOS 90, 102–3, 114–17
        type A 102
    serum
        in GH-treated hypopituitary adults 20
        in premature pubarche 90–1
        see also hyperinsulinaemia
insulin-like growth factor-I (IGF-I) 114
    misuse 120
    in premature pubarche 90, 91
    role in adrenarche 85
Internet, information for drug misusers 124
intracytoplasmic sperm injection (ICSI) 63, **64**
intrauterine insemination 63
in vitro fertilization (IVF)
    in male infertility 63
    multiple births and 60, *62*
    oocyte donation and 65
ischaemic heart disease
    in GH-deficient adults 18
    in oestrogen deficiency 26–7
    prevention **29**
isotretinoin-Roaccutane 122

Kallmann's syndrome 3–4
   male, fertility therapy 54
   ovulation induction 48
kava 120
KH 19 120
KLA-X ECM adhesion protein 4

laparoscopic ovarian diathermy (LOD) 62
legal highs 120
leptin 107–9
   discovery 107–8
   functions 108, 109, 113–14
   in humans 108–9
   mode of action 108
   patterns of obesity and 109
   receptor 108
   role in PCOS 102–3, 113
leuprolide acetate 89
LH *see* luteinizing hormone
linkage analysis 4
lipids/lipoproteins, serum
   in GH-deficient adults 18–19
   in GH-treated hypopituitary adults 20–1
   in hyperinsulinaemia 91
luteinizing hormone (LH)
   action in developing ovary 35
   β-subunit
      mutations 4
      polymorphisms 6
   in girls with irregular menses 93, 94–5, *96*, 97–8
   granulosa responses, in PCOS 115–17
   in ovulation induction 48, 49
   in PCOS progression 97–8, 114–15
   premature pubarche and 88, 89
   receptor mutations 4–5, 37
   role in ovulation 45
luteinizing hormone-releasing hormone (LHRH) *see* gonadotrophin-releasing hormone

Ma Huang 122
male infertility 4, 63–4
Medicines Control Agency 123
melatonin 123
menarche 39–44
   breast differentiation and 43–4
   disease in later life and 43
   factors affecting age at 39–40
   premature pubarche and 86, **88**
   temporal decline in age at 40
menorrhagia 40–1
menstrual cycle
   irregularity, PCOS development and 93–8
   length 41

menstruation 40–1
  duration 41
  endometrium and 41–2
metabolic stimulants 121–2
midkine (MK) 42
Misuse of Drugs Act 123
multiple pregnancy, fertility treatment and 60, *62*
myocardial infarction, in oestrogen deficiency 26–7

nalbuphine 123
'narnigens' 122
nutrition
  bone growth in adolescence and 12
  ovarian function and 113–14
nutritional supplements 120, **121**, 123

obesity
  leptin expression 108–9
  mouse models 107
  ovarian function and 114–15
ob gene
  expression in obesity 108–9
  product *see* leptin
ob/ob mice 102, 107–8
oestradiol, plasma, symptoms of oestrogen deficiency and 25
oestrogen
  deficiency 25
    adverse effects 25–8
    symptoms **29**
  endometrial angiogenesis and 41, 42
oestrogen/progesterone replacement therapy (HRT) 25–9
  advantages 25–8
  contraindications 29
  disadvantages 28–9
  indications 29
oligomenorrhoea
  anovulatory 59, *60*
  in CAH 80
  premature pubarche and 88, 89
oocytes
  donation 64–6
  freezing/maturation *in vitro* 65–6
  sources 65–6
oral contraceptive pill 42
osteocalcin, serum 13, 14
  GH therapy and 14–15
osteoporosis
  age at menarche and 43
  bone growth and 11–12
  GH replacement therapy and 21
  Japanese survey 11, *12*
  oestrogen deficiency and 25–6
  prevention **29**

ovarian cancer
  age at menarche and 43
  fertility treatment and 60–2
ovarian cycle, patterns 46
ovarian diathermy, laparoscopic (LOD) 62
ovarian dysgenesis, hypergonadotrophic (HOD) 36–7
ovarian failure 46, 64–6
  causes **64**
  fertility treatment 64–6
  osteoporosis 25
  premature, osteoporosis 25
  see also anovulation
ovarian hyperandrogenism, functional (FOH) 88–90
  predictive factors 89–90
  premature pubarche and 89
  serum insulin levels 90, 91
  triggers 90
ovarian hyperstimulation syndrome (OHSS) 60
ovary
  angiogenesis, in PCOS 103–4
  cryopreservation, in fertility management 66
  development 33–7
    endocrinological 35–6
    morphological 33–4
    stages 33, **34**
  polycystic see polycystic ovaries
  steroidogenesis, onset 35–6
  structure, in anovulatory girls 94, **95**
ovulation
  failure see anovulation
  gonadotrophic requirements 45–6
  induction 47–9, 59, 61
    complications 60–2

PCOS see polycystic ovary syndrome
peripheral arterial disease, in GH-deficient adults 17–18
Piper methysticum 120
polycystic ovaries (PCO)
  as childhood condition 101–4
  in girls with irregular menses 94–7
polycystic ovary syndrome (PCOS)
  fertility treatment 48–9, 59
    complications 60–2
    laparoscopic ovarian diathermy 62
  insulin and 102, 114–15
  leptin and 102–3, 113
  LH-β polymorphisms 6
  mechanism of anovulation 115–17
  mechanism of hyperandrogenism 90
  origin in adolescence/childhood 93–8, 101–4
  ovarian function 114–15
  premature pubarche and 86, 88, 89
  vs. non-classical CAH 80

positional cloning 4
precocious puberty
    male-limited 5, 37
    polycystic ovaries and 101
pregnancy
    adolescent 42
    termination 42
primordial germ cells 33, **34**
procaine 120
progesterone
    endometrial angiogenesis and 42
    see also oestrogen/progesterone replacement therapy
psychosexual development 71–4
    in CAH 73–4
    models 71
    prenatal hormonal model 72
psychosexual problems
    in CAH 63
    hypopituitary males 52, 53
pubarche, premature (PP) 85–91
    in CAH 85
    functional ovarian hyperandrogenism 88–90
    insulin secretion pattern 90–1
    isolated 86
    late effects 88
puberty
    complex phenotypes 5, **6**
    failure
        LH receptor mutations 4–5
        rationale for HRT 25–9
    genetics 3–6
    induction, in hypopituitary boys 52
    monogenic disorders 5, **6**
    precocious *see* precocious puberty
pyridinoline/deoxypyridinoline (PYR/DPYR), urinary **13**, 14

quality of life, in hypopituitarism 21

radiotherapy, oocyte donation after 65
5α-reductase inhibitors 122
renal cancer, age at menarche and 43

salbutamol misuse 122
season, age at menarche and 40
sex-hormone-binding globulin (SHBG) 90, 113–14, 115
sexual orientation 71
silmarin 123
smart drugs 120
sperm
    donation 64
    freezing and banking 64
sports science courses 124
stature *see* height

tamoxifen misuse 122
termination of pregnancy 42
testes
    failure 64
    sperm extraction 64
    volume, in hypogonadotrophic hypogonadism 53, 54
testosterone
    amniotic fluid, in CAH 72
    in anovulatory girls 93, *94*, 97
    in polycystic ovaries 115
    replacement, in hypopituitarism 52
thyroid hormone misuse 122
Trading Standards Authority 123
transforming growth factor $\beta1$ 42
tub **107**
Turner's syndrome
    oocyte donation 65
    osteoporosis 25, **26**
    ovarian development 34

Ultimate Orange 122
undernutrition, ovarian function in 114

valproate 123
vanadium supplements 123
vascular disease, in hypopituitarism *see* hypopituitarism, vascular disease
vascular endothelial growth factor (VEGF) 41–2, 104
venous thrombosis/embolism, HRT risks 28
virilization, female foetus 72–3

waist/hip ratio
    in GH-treated hypopituitary adults 21
    in hypopituitarism 18, **19**
weight, body
    age at menarche and 39–40
    control 107–10
    loss, in PCOS 115
    ovarian function and 113–14
    see also obesity
world wide web, information for drug misusers 124

zopiclone 123